Contents

Introduction

If you are reading this book, then you have been studying low carb diets like Keto and Carnivore, and you've heard about the benefits of fasting.

Fasting can put off many people who don't really know about it. The first thing that might come to mind when you hear the word "fasting" is a religious guru in robes going weeks without eating while living in a cave somewhere. Or you might be thinking about some kind of "detox" program where people drink lemon juice.

However, those visions are all wrong. Fasting has evolved and grown in recent years with backing from real science. Part of this trend has been the revelation that you don't need to go weeks, several days, or even 48 hours to get the full benefits of fasting.

This is even truer if you are already following a healthy low carb diet that puts you in ketosis even before fasting. However, don't worry if you're not following such a diet; intermittent fasting can help you achieve results no matter what kind of diet you're on.

In this book, we will look at a style of intermittent fasting that is both practical and achievable because you'll never go a day without eating (but you can incorporate more variations of fasting if you want to). And yet you will see many of the benefits that come from longer-term fasting programs.

So, let's get started and learn about One-Meal-a-Day Intermittent Fasting!

Chapter 1 – A Brief Overview of Nutrition

To understand why intermittent fasting works and provides the benefits it does, it is good to get a little background on nutrition. If you understand the basics first, then you will understand why low carb diets work in the first place, how they produce results similar to fasting, and finally why fasting works and enhances your weight loss and improved health that you'll see from following a low carb diet.

Quick overview: What happens when you eat

Before jumping into the specifics of low carb dieting and why it is beneficial, we need to understand what happens when you eat a "normal" meal that is largely carbohydrate based. We will begin by assuming that you have eaten a meal typical for the standard American diet, that probably derives around 50% of its calories from carbohydrates.

First off, what is a carbohydrate?

Carbohydrates are compounds that occur in food and tissues. They are made up of sugars, starches, and indigestible plant materials called "cellulose". While you might think of carbohydrates as plant-based, animals also have carbohydrates in their tissues. In animals, carbohydrates are stored in a kind of starch called *glycogen*.

Glycogen is found in two places in animals: muscle tissue and your liver. Think about it—the liver is kind of like meat but with a different texture. Part of that is due to the starch content. Of course, eating liver isn't like eating pasta or a slice of bread; in comparison, the starch content is minimal. However, if you are a carnivore who thinks you're eating a "zero carb" diet but eat some liver to get the vitamins, well, you're actually getting some carbs with it!

In muscle tissue, glycogen is used by the muscles for energy and your liver stores glycogen as a kind of sugar reserve. If you are in a situation where food isn't available, the liver will break down the glycogen into sugar and release it into the bloodstream. It does this to try and keep your blood sugar up, so you don't collapse and die or have other problems.

A key piece of info when educating yourself about low carb dieting and fasting is that while the liver stores glycogen, its capacity to do so is limited. Be sure to remember that for future reference.

So what is starch? While it is a word in common use, most people don't really know what it is. Simply put, starch is a long chain consisting of glucose molecules hooked together. In other words, starch is nothing more than sugar. It's considered a little healthier by the nutrition "experts" because it takes a little longer to digest than pure sugar because your body has to break it apart into the individual sugars first. But in the end, it is nothing more than sugar.

Plants contain carbohydrates in the form of cellulose that is indigestible to humans. It usually goes by another name on food labels: fiber or dietary fiber. Fiber can help you since it aids with digestion and keeping stools firm and moving through at a regular rate. A lack of fiber in your diet can cause constipation and even diarrhea. Carnivore dieters who absolutely reject plants can experience much constipation and diarrhea in the early phases of their diet since their body has to adjust to a lack of fiber.

When it comes to everything else—bread, pasta, "whole grains", potatoes, oranges, apples, or bananas—the bottom line is these are all sugar based foods. No matter what differences there are between them, in the end, they are all sugar.

The speed at which the sugar enters your system varies depending on how complex the molecule is that the sugar is stored in ("complex carbohydrates") and the fiber content of the food. The simpler the food, the faster it will make your blood sugar rise, and your blood sugar will probably rise to a higher peak.

Nutrition scientists have tried to package these differences into a measurement called the "glycemic index". It is a kind of score that ranks foods on how badly they impact blood sugar. The score ranges from 1-100, with 1 being something that barely impacts blood sugar—if at all—and 100 being pure glucose. The glycemic index has been used to keep people with metabolic problems (pre-diabetics and type 2 diabetics) eating carbohydrates. Some people simply can't let carbohydrates go. In any case, if a food has a glycemic index of 55 or less, it's considered to have a low glycemic index. Moderate ranges are between 56-69, and high is 70+.

Let's look at some examples. Non-starchy vegetables like leafy greens have a glycemic index of 15 or less, which makes them very low. Put another way; they barely impact blood sugar—if at all. That is why you can eat all the leafy greens you want on a keto diet. However, watch out for starchy vegetables, even if they are green. While broccoli has a glycemic index of 10, green peas have a glycemic index of 48, higher than many fruits. Bell peppers have a glycemic index of 15, similar to spinach.

A fruit like an orange checks in at 43-59 (depending on the type). Even though oranges contain a lot of sugar, they have a relatively low glycemic index because of the fiber content of the fruit. Not all fruit fares so well; dates have a glycemic index of 100. Compare an orange to orange juice, which checks in at 71. Same ingredients but without the fiber, so it is easier for your body to digest the orange juice leading to a faster rise in blood sugar.

Enter Insulin

Now let's say you have eaten some starchy food and it has been broken down into the sugar components. The sugar enters the bloodstream, then what happens?

Your pancreas detects this and releases a hormone called insulin. You have probably heard much about insulin, especially in relation to diabetics. Cells can use sugar for energy, but they need insulin to get it. Insulin basically allows sugar to enter the cells.

Insulin is a natural substance made by the pancreas, but it can also be given as a medication for those who either can't make insulin or can't make enough of it to be effective.

Type 1 diabetics have a chronic condition whereby their bodies make either no insulin at all or only trace amounts. They have to be given insulin by injection every time they eat for the rest of their lives. Type 2 diabetics have problems with insulin due to the system wearing out. They may or may not need insulin injections, and it is possible that different diets can help type 2 diabetics get off insulin and other medications.

So insulin acts like a key that opens a door in your cells so they can take up the blood sugar and use it for energy. But that isn't all insulin does.

The cells will only take up so much blood sugar. In other words, they will take up what they need to satisfy energy requirements. Something has to be done with the excess blood sugar. And when you understand that, you'll understand why people get fat.

Insulin has two more jobs to do. The first is to get the liver to store whatever blood sugar is left over. The liver will start doing this by repackaging the glucose into starch molecules—the starch called glycogen that we talked about earlier. And you should remember that the liver's capacity to store glycogen is limited. So, suppose it's already at maximum capacity? What happens then?

Then the liver starts repackaging the sugar into fat molecules. Pretty interesting, isn't it, that the body can do something like that? The liver can also store fat, but again has a limited capacity to do so. And having a lot of fat in your liver isn't healthy; there is a condition called "fatty liver". In any case, when the liver can't make and store fat, it releases it into the bloodstream. Now insulin has another job to do.

Insulin's other job is to get fat cells to take up and store that fat. The good or bad news is that fat cells have basically unlimited capacity for fat storage. So if you are getting excess calories over time, it's going to cause your body to store more energy as fat in your fat cells.

In the modern world, where food is cheap, plentiful, and readily available, and most of us are living sedentary lifestyles, this can be a troublesome thing. It is why so many of us are overweight or obese. Fat tissue is called "adipose" tissue by professionals.

However, in the grand scheme of things, storing a lot of body fat is a good thing! In times when food isn't available, that body fat provides a reservoir of energy to keep you from starving to death! Under the right circumstances, your body will release the fat from the fat cells so you can burn it for energy.

As we will see, that is where intermittent fasting comes in (and it has other benefits too).

Glucagon

While insulin gets all the press, there is another important hormone your body uses related to the system just described: glucagon. Like insulin, glucagon is made by the pancreas. Also, like insulin, glucagon is important in the maintenance of blood sugar levels, but it acts in opposite ways to insulin.

Remember: insulin promotes the manufacture of glycogen from glucose in the liver; glucagon does the opposite. When the pancreas releases glucagon, it promotes the breakdown of glycogen in the liver into individual glucose molecules that are released into the bloodstream, keeping blood sugar up.

Like insulin, glucagon is also available as an injectable medication. It can be used in a hypoglycemic emergency (very low blood sugar) to raise blood sugar levels in a patient.

Glucagon has another task. Remember that insulin causes fat made by the liver to be stored in fat cells. Glucagon does the opposite—it tells fat cells to release fat into the bloodstream so that it can be used for energy.

Let's summarize.

Insulin does the following:

- Tells cells to take up sugar after a meal.
- Tells the liver to make left-over sugar into glycogen.
- When the liver has stored all the glycogen and fat it can, it tells fat cells to take up the left-over fat molecules made by the liver and store them.

We can summarize all those like this: insulin tries to lower blood sugar, and it promotes the storage of glycogen and body fat.

Glucagon:

- Tells the liver to break down glycogen into sugar molecules and raise blood sugar.
- It promotes the release of fat from fat cells.

So glucagon tries to raise blood sugar and promotes the release of body fat for energy use. We can say that insulin and glucagon have a yin-yang relationship. This relationship between the two hormones is something we can exploit by fasting.

Insulin Resistance

Think about the first time you rode a roller coaster. It seemed really scary, and your stomach was filled with butterflies at every turn.

However, if you keep riding the roller coaster, each time you do it, you will experience less and less fear. That happens at a gut level too, no more butterflies, and eventually it might get boring if you keep riding it.

The same thing happens with insulin in many people. Their cells become less responsive to the lock and key effect of insulin. In other words, insulin tries to get the cells to take up the sugar in your blood, but over time, they get used to insulin and start getting less responsive to its presence.

This is called insulin resistance.

Another side of the same coin is insulin sensitivity, a measure of how sensitive your body is in carrying out the jobs insulin wants it to carry out.

People who are pre-diabetic or diabetic, or on their way down that path, suffer from insulin resistance. Now, remember that getting the cells to take up blood sugar is only one of the jobs insulin has; it also promotes the manufacture of glycogen in the liver and tells fat cells to store fat.

If a person has insulin resistance, there are a few things that happen:

- Since cells aren't as responsive when it comes to taking up blood sugar, the blood sugar level rises. A person might feel a little fatigued since the cells aren't getting enough fuel.
- If nothing else changes, the liver stored all the glycogen it could already.
- So the body begins making fat, and insulin gets the fat cells to take it up. Weight gain ensues.

Oh, and one more thing happens. In an effort to try harder to get the cells to take up the blood sugar, the pancreas makes and releases more insulin into the bloodstream. That is why the insulin level in your blood is one marker for health your doctor might be interested in. Higher insulin levels can cause even more weight gain (more insulin → more food energy stored as fat). Eventually, the pancreas can wear out, and so after a lot of damage has been done, it can't make enough insulin for the body to function properly. In other words, you have developed diabetes. High insulin levels can also cause imbalances in blood lipids (cholesterol, HDL/good cholesterol, triglycerides).

As we will see, fasting is a powerful tool you can use to keep your insulin system working properly. It can also heal a defective metabolism.

One Body – Two States

You may be noticing that glucagon is a hormone that acts on the body to get it to provide its own sources of energy, whether that is by causing the liver to break down glycogen and release blood sugar or whether it's getting fat cells to release fat. You have also learned that insulin works to get food energy (from carbs) into your cells and helps the excess get stored in reserves, whether that's in the form of sugar stored in the liver as glycogen or by promoting storage of body fat.

So we see two states the body can be in when it comes to food:

> • The fed state: food energy is coming in. Insulin acts to promote its use and storage.
> • The fasting state: glucagon takes over, and acts to break down stored food energy so the body can use it.

Therefore, fasting isn't some weird, unusual thing; it is a natural part of the body's functioning. You fast all the time already. The most obvious point of fasting is when you sleep. Depending on when your last meal was, and the first time of day you typically eat, you've fasted anywhere from eight-twelve hours.

That is why the first meal of the day was traditionally called breakfast—it literally means to break (or end) fast.

We also see a relationship between insulin and glucagon:

> • Insulin levels high, glucagon levels low.

- Glucagon levels high, insulin levels low.

By voluntarily fasting for longer periods than simply sleeping overnight, we can promote more usage of glucagon that helps break down stored food energy, leading to more weight loss and better long-term health.

Grazing and Eating Throughout the Day

Besides promoting low-fat, high-carb eating patterns, one of the worst things the medical and nutritional establishments have done over the past 50 years is to promote the nonsensical idea of "grazing". This is the idea that rather than eating three large meals, you should eat four, five, or even six smaller meals spread evenly throughout the day. All low fat, of course.

If you are eating six low-fat meals during your waking hours, knowing what you know now about insulin, what is your take on how this situation will play out?

You are going to be chronically in a fed state. And when you're in a fed state—and continually taking in more carbs all day long—you're promoting insulin release.

The experts thought the good thing about having six meals a day was it would prevent blood sugar crashes. Well, maybe that is true, as your blood sugar drops from the last meal you had, then you eat more carbs and get it back up again. However, you are continually having insulin do its job, and part of that job is to tell fat cells to take up and store more fat.

Some people might do OKAY eating six meals a day, but it is hard to see how keeping insulin going full bore the entire waking day is a great idea.

Suppose instead that we ate fewer carbs—giving insulin less to do so that your pancreas will release less of it into the bloodstream? And suppose that we ate less often so that we could strengthen this effect?

That sounds better than eating carbs all day long if optimum health is one of your goals.

Metabolic Disorder

Diabetes is a serious public health issue. Tens of millions of people in the United States have it, and tens of millions more have "pre-diabetes", a condition where blood sugars are getting higher but not high enough to indicate diabetes. Diabetes is deadly serious. A person with diabetes is far more likely to have a heart attack, stroke, and even cancer—and that can happen even with treatment! Left untreated, diabetics can also develop blindness, suffer from kidney damage, and have poor wound healing that can lead to serious infections and even amputation. Many of these health problems arise because high blood sugar, when chronic and going through high spikes, can damage blood vessels. When tissue and organs like your kidneys or limbs don't get a good blood supply, they get damaged.

Over the past twenty years, doctors have begun to put together a picture like a jigsaw puzzle. There are many health problems you can think of that seem to be related to "middle age". These include:

- Weight gain, often around the midsection.
- High blood sugar.
- High cholesterol.
- Low HDL or "good" cholesterol.
- High blood pressure.
- High triglycerides—a type of blood fat associated with an increased risk of heart attack and stroke. It turns out that high triglycerides are caused by too much sugar and starch in the diet.

The stereotype of this is the man with the "beer belly". You can have a "beer belly" without drinking beer because the condition isn't so much from beer in particular as it is from the starches that are in the beer. So, eating any kind of carb-based diet puts you at risk as the years go by.

Medical professionals noticed that these health issues—while each can occur in isolation—usually arise in a cluster. Typically, a person will have three or more of them, and quite often suffer from all of these problems. This is called metabolic syndrome.

Metabolic syndrome is considered to be a defect in the metabolism—specifically, it is related to the digestion of carbohydrates. Whether it's really a defect or not depends on your perspective. Those who consider it a defect believe that eating a carbohydrate-based diet is natural, healthy, and desirable. This point of view is questionable. What if instead, since our ancestors lived through eons of time when animal protein was the dominant food source, a carbohydrate-based diet is, in fact, unnatural and undesirable? Maybe people with metabolic syndrome don't really have a syndrome at all—maybe high amounts of carbohydrates in the diet is akin to eating poison. And maybe people who don't get metabolic syndrome are simply more adept at handling the poison.

Doctors, being doctors, will approach the problem of metabolic syndrome in a predictable fashion. First, they will say, "Diet and exercise." The primary problem with this is that "diet" to them actually means to eat more carbohydrates! They will tell you to eat "fruit and "whole grains." While a whole grain food is harder to digest—and so won't raise blood sugar as rapidly and maybe not as high—, you are still eating a sugar-based diet if you follow this advice. Second, if one's diet is not properly addressed, while exercise has many benefits not related to weight loss, exercise alone is not going to cure metabolic syndrome.

This brings our medical friends to the inevitable end game—which is to load up their patients on medications. First, it might start with high blood pressure pills, and pills to control triglyceride levels and cholesterol. By now, the patient is trapped in an endless cycle. Eventually, for many, diabetes will be the result. Then, more pills, and for some, insulin injections. Plus, despite all this, health problems are probably down the road, including a heart attack. But doctors will say it was "inevitable" and "can only get worse," and the best they can do is "control it."

Two natural cures can reverse metabolic syndrome and avoid the above scenario. They are:

- Follow a low-carb diet.
- Incorporate intermittent fasting into your lifestyle.

Now a quick primer on blood lipids for those who need a review, and to understand fasting properly.

Blood Lipids

"Blood lipids" are fat and fat-containing molecules transported by the bloodstream. The most famous blood lipid is cholesterol. Your body needs cholesterol despite all the bad press it has had. It's used to make hormones and provides structural components for cell membranes. Cholesterol is transported through the bloodstream by two different molecules. The first is called LDL or "bad" cholesterol. LDL means "low-density lipoprotein". LDL isn't really cholesterol; it is a molecule used to transport it to the various body tissues (it contains cholesterol). Lipoprotein means fat + protein.

LDL cholesterol can cause heart disease by sticking to artery walls. Depending on the components in the diet, it can be small and hard or large and fluffy. If you eat a carbohydrate-based diet, LDL particles get small and hard, and they can stick to artery walls, which eventually leads to blockages causing a heart attack and/or stroke. However, if you eat a fat-based low-carb diet, your LDL particles will get large and fluffy, and they are far less likely to stick to artery walls. Hence eating a low carb diet can reduce the risk of heart disease.

The other kind of cholesterol you have probably heard about is "good cholesterol". This is high-density lipoprotein or HDL. The main job of HDL appears to be to act as a clean-up crew. It gathers up excess LDL and, apparently, even LDL stuck to your artery walls and returns it to the liver. The higher your HDL, the lower your risk of heart disease and stroke.

The final blood lipid of note is triglycerides. Doctors didn't really take triglycerides too seriously until recently. Remember how many decades passed when all they talked about was total cholesterol? Then, for a while, it was good and bad cholesterol. Well, now it is good and bad cholesterol and triglycerides.

It turns out that high triglycerides are a marker of bad health. Basically:

- A fasting triglyceride level of above 149 mg/dL is bad.
- A fasting triglyceride level of 100-149 is considered "normal", but it's not great.
- A fasting triglyceride level of less than 100 is ideal.

It turns out that triglyceride levels and HDL cholesterol levels tend to be paired in opposite ways:

- People with high triglycerides usually have low HDL cholesterol.
- People with low triglycerides tend to have high HDL cholesterol.

So, triglycerides are tied very closely to a heart attack risk:

- High triglycerides (above 149 mg/dL) and low HDL (below 40 mg/dL) is tied to a very high risk of having a heart attack in the future.
- Low triglycerides (especially below 100) and high HDL (at least 45, over 50 desirable) is tied to a very low risk of having a heart attack in the future.

The medical establishment still goes around peddling the lie that high triglycerides are caused by eating a fatty diet. This is completely false.

High triglycerides are caused by:

- Eating carbohydrates.

- High insulin levels.
- To some extent, family history.

So, guess what—people who are prone to diabetes usually have high triglycerides and low HDL cholesterol. This is true whether or not you have developed diabetes yet.

However, guess what cures a high triglyceride level? Of course, doctors are anxious to put you on prescription medications for it, but there are two natural ways you can do it without their help:

- High fish oil doses.
- Eat a low-carb diet.

Oh, and one more way to help lower triglycerides—intermittent fasting.

Summary

In this chapter, we have reviewed the role played by the two digestive related hormones that regulate blood sugar, glycogen storage, and body fat. These hormones are insulin and glucagon. Insulin is a hormone related to the "fed" state—when you eat, insulin is released into the bloodstream to encourage cells to take up blood sugar that they can use for energy. Some blood sugar will be left over, and insulin promotes the manufacture of glycogen or stored starch in the liver. If the capacity for glycogen in the liver has been maximized, the liver will make fat instead. If the capacity for fat storage by the liver has been maxed out, the fat will be released into the bloodstream and insulin prompts fat cells to take it up and store it. So, insulin can help make people fat, and this happens when people eat many carbohydrates.

Glucagon operates in the fasting state—when the body has been without food for a while. It promotes the breakdown of glycogen in the liver into glucose to keep blood sugars up. Glucagon also promotes the release of fat by the fat cells to use as energy.

People can become insulin resistant—meaning their cells don't respond when insulin tries to get them to take up sugar. The pancreas responds by making and releasing more insulin. This can lead to more weight gain and a vicious cycle of increasing insulin resistance that can lead to diabetes, and the pancreas wears out and isn't as able to make enough insulin to keep up. People with type 2 diabetes or heading that way will develop high blood sugars—since the sugar isn't being properly utilized by the body's cells.

Metabolic syndrome results when a person develops high blood sugar, belly fat, high blood triglycerides, high cholesterol, low HDL or good cholesterol, and possibly high blood pressure.

People who have diabetes often have metabolic syndrome. Diabetics and people with metabolic syndrome are at high risk for having a heart attack and/or stroke.

The basket of problems associated with metabolic syndrome, including weight gain, can be treated naturally by the adaptation of a low-carb diet. Any low-carb type of lifestyle is helpful, but the keto diet appears to be the best diet suited for this purpose. Moreover, fasting, which acts on the body in similar ways to a keto diet, is an option that can help people enhance the benefits they can achieve by following a low-carb lifestyle.

In the following chapters, we will review the phenomenon of ketosis and provide an overview of low-carb dieting options. Ketosis is a process by which the body utilizes fat rather than sugar for energy. When it comes to low carb, it is important to realize that low-carb eating is not really dieting per se, even if losing weight is the goal of many people. Low carb is more like a lifestyle change than a diet, and when you reach your weight loss goals, it is good to stay on low carb for the long haul. This will result in a healthy, adjusted metabolic system.

Chapter 2 – An Introduction to Ketosis and Intermittent Fasting

Now that you have a basic understanding of what happens when you digest food, you can begin to look at fasting and how it can help with weight loss and improving health overall. Before getting into the details of intermittent fasting, we will discuss ketosis, which is burning fat for energy. The reason this will be discussed is that all types of fasting rely on ketosis. An overview of the different styles or methods of fasting is also provided.

What is Ketosis?

In the last chapter, you learned about what happens when you digest carbohydrates and how your body responds to glucose in your bloodstream with insulin. Under normal circumstances when you are consuming carbohydrates, the body will utilize the sugar for energy. It can be said that burning carbohydrates for energy is the basic or default state of the body. This is not because burning carbohydrates for energy is better—it's not; it is just easier to burn carbohydrates. However, fat produces more energy. Each gram of carbohydrates produces four calories of energy, whereas a gram of fat produces more than twice as much at nine calories.

When the supply of carbohydrates in the body is low, the body breaks down fat into molecules called *ketones* that it can use for energy. Ketones are made from fat in the liver and released into the bloodstream where they can be transported to the body's cells, including your brain, which then uses them for energy. The process of using ketones for energy is called ketosis.

There are many ways that you can get your body into ketosis. One undesirable method is through starvation. With no carbohydrates available, a person that is starving has no options—their body will use ketosis to get energy for as long as it can after the glycogen stores have been exhausted in the liver.

Remember that glycogen is a kind of starch that is stored in your liver to use as an emergency reserve. When there isn't any other source of glucose available, then the liver will break down the glycogen into individual glucose molecules so that the blood glucose level will be kept within a healthy range. However, this procedure only works for a short time. The liver only has enough glycogen for this process to last about 24 hours.

People with diabetes can also enter a state where the body has ketones in the bloodstream in an involuntary fashion. This occurs when the patient has an inadequate level of insulin or misses doses. This will lead to the patient entering a state called ketoacidosis, where blood sugar is extremely high, there are ketones in the blood, and the blood becomes acidic. This is an emergency situation and not to be confused with the state of ketosis. When you are in a state of ketosis, your blood is not acidic. A diabetic in ketoacidosis will experience mental confusion, frequent urination, nausea, and vomiting. It is usually treated by the administration of insulin and is more common among type 1 diabetics.

Ketosis is a completely natural state. It is the body's healthy reaction to the unavailability of glucose as a fuel.

There are three ways that you can enter a state of ketosis on purpose. One way is through exercise, but that is not the most efficient method. You can also enter ketosis by following a low-carb diet. The third way is by fasting, which is the voluntary deprivation of food, but for a fixed time.

What is Intermittent Fasting?

Previously you learned that being in the fed state can cause many health problems. Insulin levels remain high, which leads to weight gain and insulin resistance. Over the long term, this can lead to the development of health problems, including diabetes, inflammation, heart disease, and even cancer.

Intermittent fasting is going without food for a fixed period on purpose. This is done to promote the fasting state, where the hormone glucagon acts to promote weight loss. And when this happens, insulin levels are reduced. As a result, the body can experience the following changes:

- Reduced blood sugars.

- Increased insulin sensitivity—or put another way, decreased insulin resistance.

- Smaller glycogen stores in the liver.

- Smaller fat stores in the liver.

- Your body spends more time burning its fat for energy, resulting in healthy weight loss.

- Fasting promotes an increase in human growth hormone.

- The process of *autophagy* is triggered, renewing the body's cells and tissues, slowing the aging process and promoting overall health.

To summarize, intermittent fasting promotes a reduction in insulin and blood sugar, human growth hormone and autophagy, while helping to repair disorders in the metabolism. It may be the case that intermittent fasting can increase lifespan.

Extended Fasting

It is possible to fast for an extended period, from more than one day to several days to weeks. Some people claim additional health benefits, but this is not to be confused with intermittent fasting.

Types of Intermittent Fasting

There are many different ways that you can implement intermittent fasting. The term intermittent means *occurring at periodic intervals, not continuous or steady*. Hence, we are not talking about fasting for 40 days and 40 nights in a row. Intermittent fasting means picking a regular slot in your calendar to fast for a limited time. When you practice intermittent fasting, periods where your body is in the fed state are decreased. This is done to limit or minimize the time during which insulin is acting on the body and all that comes along with it. Intermittent fasting can be done on a personalized basis.

In short, intermittent fasting means *time restricting food intake,* and in many cases, is not technically "fasting", which involves going at least 24 hours without consuming food.

When you utilize intermittent fasting, your day or week will be broken up into a *fasting* period, and a *feeding* period. The fasting period will be either a time frame where you only consume water or beverages, like coffee, tea, or bone broth that are either zero calories or negligible calories—although some methods of fasting allow the consumption of a minimal number of calories.

Fasting has a long history behind it going back to ancient times. It was long recognized as a method of healing the body and promoting health and has been used as a tool to achieve mental clarity and attain spiritual insights by the world's great religious traditions. Hippocrates, the Ancient Greek physician, was one of the first medical practitioners to note that fasting was a way to help the body heal itself. However, the benefits of fasting were lost to history in recent centuries when the wider availability of food led people astray, focusing on eating all the time rather than experiencing the benefits of fasting. This all changed with the introduction of the 5:2 diet.

Let's examine the most popular methods of intermittent fasting:

The 5:2 Diet

Intermittent fasting is fasting that you do on a scheduled, regular basis that is time-limited. One way that you can do this, and that became very popular a few years back, is to fast two days per week, and eat normally five days per week. This type of fasting is called the 5:2 diet. Although you can use the 5:2 diet with keto or a paleo lifestyle, no specific method of dieting is required. You can even use the 5:2 fasting with the standard American diet if you want to.

When following the 5:2 diet, the two fasting days must be separated by at least one day of eating. So eating Monday, Wednesday, Friday, Saturday, and Sunday, while fasting on Tuesday and Thursday would be acceptable. However, fasting Tuesday and Wednesday while eating the remaining days would not be.

On the fasting days, there are two options. The first is to actually fast, which means only consuming calorie-free liquids. The second option is to engage in calorie restriction on the fasting day. Using this method, you still eat on a fasting day, but you limit your total caloric intake to 500 calories.

The 4:3 Diet

The 4:3 diet uses the same principles of the 5:2 diet, but adds in one more day of fasting. As with the 5:2 diet, the three fasting days must be separated from each other by at least one day where the body is in a fed state, and fasting days can either be actual fasting or simply reduced-calorie days.

Full 24-Hour Fasting sometimes called "Eat Stop Eat"

One of the most basic ways to fast is to avoid eating for a straight 24-hour period, and then eat again. This basic type of one day fast was called "Eat Stop Eat" in a book written by Brad Pilon. This type of fasting takes more discipline and is not for everyone.

48-Hour Fast

This is an extension of full 24-hour fasting into two days.

Extended Fasting

As you can see, we can continue the process by adding more days to the fasting. A program of extended fasting involves fasting for at least three days and up to seven days. When following a program of extended fasting, the fasting days all occur right in a row. This is a more extreme version of fasting and not recommended.

Dry Fasting

Dry fasting is a variant of a 24-hour or 48-hour fast where liquids are also avoided.

Alternate Day Fasting

Alternate day fasting is another way to describe 4:3 fasting. It is simply fasting one day and eating the next, then fasting again, with up to three fasting days per week allowed.

Warrior Diet

The warrior diet is a method of fasting that can be incorporated into the lifestyles of people who utilize intense, vigorous exercise. This is a method of fasting that uses one large meal per day. The general plan is to engage in vigorous exercise twenty hours after your last meal, and then you eat the next large meal within four hours of your exercise session.

Fasting Mimicking Diet

The fasting mimicking diet, or FMD, involves picking out between two-five days per month where a reduced-calorie diet is consumed. On reduced-calorie days, a diet of 800-1,000 calories per day is allowed. In that sense, it is not a true fasting diet. On fasting days, the participant is supposed to eat low-calorie foods that are moderate in protein, fat, and carbohydrates. Common examples include mushrooms and olives. This type of diet has been shown to reduce insulin and blood pressure.

One-Meal-a-Day Fasting

This is the main focus of this book. Using this method, you eat one meal per day—generally recommended two-three days per week if you are following a diet that already puts you in ketosis like keto or Atkins. If you are not following any specialized diet, you can utilize one-meal-a-day fasting daily. That will help ensure that you spend a lot of time in ketosis no matter what you are eating.

16:8 Fasting

This type of fasting limits the fed state to eight hours each day while fasting the other sixteen hours. For example, you can restrict your eating from ten a.m. to six p.m., or eleven a.m. to seven p.m. Advocates of a 16:8 hour fast suggest that you set a goal of eating your last meal of the day before seven p.m., and the evidence shows that this leads to better outcomes. You can use 16:8 fasting daily, or just a few days per week.

20:4 Fasting

As the name suggests, this is a variation of the 16:8 fasting plan. The time spent fasting is increased to twenty hours per day, and the eating window or fed state is limited to four hours. You can eat one or two meals using this type of fasting; for example, you can eat between two p.m. and six p.m. each day. Like 16:8 fasting, you can do this frequently, even every single day, if you want to.

Starvation vs. Fasting

Many people confuse starvation mode with fasting; however, they are not the same. The first obvious difference is that when the body is in starvation mode, this is an involuntary state. Maybe there has been a famine where all the crops were destroyed or perhaps you have been taken prisoner. The exact reason isn't important; the point is some outside force is preventing you from obtaining food you want to eat.

However, that is not the only difference. Even when a person is entering a state of starvation, they initially go through a state of fasting. In short, fasting is a state of utilizing the body's stored fat for energy to get through a short period where food isn't available. This developed in prehistoric times when people had to have energy available to function in between being able to hunt or gather food. Your body also goes into a fasting state each night when you sleep, as discussed in the previous chapter. In other words, when you are in the fasting state, you're going to be obtaining food in short order, whether it is later in the day, the following day, or a couple of days from now. When you are in a starvation state, you may not ever get adequate food. Starvation doesn't necessarily involve the complete absence of calories either; you could be getting a level of calories that is below subsistence levels.

When the body is in fasting mode, it will maintain normal levels of metabolism. When the body enters starvation mode, which happens when there is a prolonged absence of adequate calories, the body will massively slow down its metabolism to conserve energy. Eventually, the body will begin to devour itself, consuming its muscle tissue for the protein content, and it will be malnourished due to the lack of proper vitamins, minerals, and other nutrients.

The Benefits of Intermittent Fasting

As touched on earlier, there are many benefits of intermittent fasting. People seeking to improve their health, especially those who are suffering from pre-diabetes, obesity, or even diabetes, will benefit immensely from the reduction in insulin levels and blood sugar. There are many options available for fasting, and you can personalize it to your lifestyle and diet:

- Reduction in blood sugar. When you are fasting, one obvious consequence is that you're not consuming carbohydrates. Blood sugar levels will drop and be maintained at a lower level.

- Reduction in insulin levels. Studies show that while fasting, insulin levels will drop. In fact, we know this from first principles—since insulin levels rise in response to the intake of food (carbohydrates) and decrease in response to the fasting state.

- Weight loss. Intermittent fasting will help you lose weight. In the short term, depriving the body of calories will rev up the metabolism.

- Reduction in belly fat. Fasting appears to be very beneficial for people who have metabolic syndrome. One of the results of incorporating a fasting program into your lifestyle is a reduction in belly fat.

- Reduced triglycerides. Fasting can reduce blood triglycerides since they are primarily produced in response to the consumption of carbohydrates or alcohol.

- Renewal of the body's tissues. Intermittent fasting promotes autophagy and an increase in human growth hormone.

- Reduced risk of heart disease. In recent years, doctors have realized that high blood sugars and high triglycerides are among the most important factors in determining a person's risk for contracting heart disease. By reducing insulin, blood sugar, and triglycerides, fasting can help reduce the risk of both having a heart attack and stroke.

- Reduced risk of diabetes. Intermittent fasting reduces insulin levels during the fasting period, and this helps the body increase insulin sensitivity. With increased insulin sensitivity, there will be lower blood sugars. The amazing thing about the increased insulin sensitivity produced by intermittent fasting is that this helps in general so that even if you are consuming some carbohydrates as part of your normal diet, your body will handle them better in a healthier fashion because insulin resistance is reduced. In some cases, diabetes can even be reversed.

The Impact of Fasting on IGF-1

IGF-1 is a growth hormone called "insulin-like growth factor one". This hormone has many effects; some good, some bad. Among the bad, IGF-1 may promote the growth of cancer and reduce lifespan. IGF-1 helps maintain normal blood sugar levels but has a relatively weak impact as compared to insulin. It can promote normal cell growth and is also involved in the mediation of the effects of human growth hormone. It has been found that at least some types of fasting can reduce levels of IGF-1. Although the hormone has some positive effects, it is generally considered a good thing to lower IGF-1 levels in the blood.

Who Should Not Fast

Intermittent fasting sounds easy, practical, and beneficial. And for the vast majority of people, it is. However, it is important to recognize that intermittent fasting is not for everyone. You should speak to your doctor if you plan to incorporate fasting into your lifestyle, but there are certain groups of people that need to be extra cautious about taking up fasting if they indeed take it up at all. Let's quickly review people who are not going to be well suited to fasting:

- New mothers, especially if they are breastfeeding. New moms should not take up fasting. If a woman is breastfeeding, fasting is out of the question during this temporary situation.

- Pregnant women. A woman should not fast during pregnancy as she needs to maintain high levels of nutritional food consumption to ensure that the fetus develops normally.
- Anyone suffering from anorexia or bulimia. If you are suffering from a food or eating-related disorder, please seek the help of your doctor. In no case should anyone who is suffering from anorexia or bulimia consider fasting.
- Type 1 Diabetics.
- Type 2 Diabetics. Type 2 diabetics can take up fasting but need to do so under medical supervision. Fasting may result in unusually low blood sugars, and in all cases, will possibly require the adjustment of your medications. Anyone diagnosed as a type 2 diabetic needs to speak to their doctor before beginning a fasting program.
- Pre-diabetics. While pre-diabetics may not have to worry about medication, they should approach fasting with care. If you are not following a keto diet, low blood sugars may result, risking hypoglycemia. If you are already on prescription medication, like metformin, you must speak to your doctor about incorporating fasting into your lifestyle.
- People under the age of eighteen. Anyone who is under the age of eighteen should not engage in fasting, even if endorsed by parents.
- The elderly. Anyone who is elderly should not fast unless it can be done under a reasonable level of supervision.
- Thin people. If your BMI is lower than what is considered normal, then you should not fast.

A word of caution to people who are not in any of the above categories: When you take up fasting for the first few times, do so under very controlled circumstances in case problems arise. Try it a few times before you decide to fast and engage in any vigorous physical activity, and ease into your physical workout routine a few times before going full steam ahead.

Who is Fasting For?

Fasting is virtually for anyone who is not on the previous list. If you are obese or overweight, then fasting is definitely something you can incorporate into your health and weight loss program, provided that you are not a diagnosed diabetic on insulin or other medications. Fasting will definitely help you normalize your blood sugars, lose weight, reduce your blood pressure, and lower your triglycerides, among other benefits.

Fasting can also be incorporated into your lifestyle if you are not overweight or obese but are simply seeking to maximize your health. Many people who are in normal weight ranges do exactly this. Fasting will help you maintain your weight and good health over time. Fasting can also help you avoid diabetes by keeping insulin levels low and encouraging heightened insulin sensitivity. In addition, there are many other benefits that you can realize from fasting that aren't related to weight loss or health related to blood sugar.

In any case, if you have any known health difficulties or encounter any problems while fasting, you should consult with your doctor.

How long do you need to fast and why?

There are two main goals of fasting you should be conscious of along with the time required to achieve both:

> • Burning through glycogen stores: The first goal of fasting is to get through the glycogen stores in the liver. The reason we do this is so that we can put the body in a state of ketosis. If you are already following a low-carb or keto diet, then you may have already done this. It takes at least six-eight hours to get through your glycogen stores and start burning fat. You can see why eating late at night, and then again first thing in the morning causes problems with weight gain or inhibiting weight loss—there isn't much, if any, time to burn off fat if

you follow that type of eating pattern. Also, constant "grazing" throughout the day means the stores of glycogen in the liver will be constantly replenished.

• Autophagy: If you are incorporating fasting in your lifestyle for health, you will want to fast long enough to trigger autophagy. At a minimum, it will take twelve-sixteen hours to trigger this.

So we see that at the bare minimum it will take twelve hours to enter a fasted state, and research assumes this. Studies of men following a fasted diet pattern with a twelve-hour window of eating didn't show any benefits. The reason is that having a twelve-hour window during which you consume food means that you eat immediately just as you are entering the fasted state.

The same studies found that participants did accrue a large number of benefits from limiting eating to an eight-hour window. This puts the total time without eating at sixteen hours per day, and the time in the truly fasted state at about four hours. So, the 16:8 plan will give you a small amount of time fasting each day, which will certainly help. It was found that even if there was no weight loss, participants that fasted with a 16:8 method showed other benefits, such as lowered blood pressure, lower blood sugar, and lowered triglycerides.

Chapter 3 – One-Meal-A-Day Intermittent Fasting: The Basics

The 16:8 fasting method has much appeal to people who are looking for a way to fast without skipping an entire day before their next meal. However, as you saw at the end of the last chapter, the benefits from fasting are at a bare minimum when following this pattern. There simply is not enough time in the fasted state for the body to get the benefits. It is a straightforward matter to observe from this that we can start shrinking the window during which you consume food in order to increase the benefits your body can achieve from fasting while still being able to eat every day. This might be something that you wish to pursue; you can have a personalized window of eating that could be six hours, or four hours rather than a full eight-hour window. However, if you are going to eat over four hours or less, it makes more sense to eat one large meal rather than trying to fit one or more meals into a short timespan like four hours.

What is the One-Meal-A-Day Intermittent Fasting Diet?

Naturally, carrying out this reduction process leads you to eat one meal per day with no consumption "window" at all. A limiting process that continually shrinks the consumption window can be applied, while still maintaining the goal of getting food every day. In other words, why not simply eat just once every twenty-four hours?

The principles of the one-meal-a-day approach are very straightforward. You simply follow these rules:

> • Fasting period: You fast for 23 hours each day. During this time, you only consume liquids that have zero or very little calories. Most people will limit themselves to water and perhaps tea or coffee. It's important to note if you choose to drink tea or coffee that they are diuretics, and keeping up your water consumption during fasting is important. In addition, some people will drink bone broth while fasting, which may provide a small number of calories. However, the calories in bone broth can be considered negligible, and people are drinking bone broth to get the mineral content and not for calories.
>
> • Eating period: You consume your one meal a day in a time window of 60 minutes or less.

Eating one meal a day has more benefits than first meets the eye. Certainly, doing so will give you a larger amount of time in the actual fasted state than what you will get having a large consumption window of up to eight hours. However, there is a second benefit in that you are going to be consuming less food. You can have a large meal during your 60-minute window, but there is only so much you can eat in one sitting even if you gorge yourself. As a result, your total caloric intake will be reduced even if you're eating a large amount during your meal as compared to following a 16:8 type of intermittent fasting.

Scientific research has shown that reduced-calorie diets can increase longevity while slowing down the aging process. However, a reduced-calorie diet comes with some downsides. People who follow a reduced-calorie diet find that they have less energy, feel cold, and have a lower libido. Typically, a person following a reduced-calorie diet will limit their total calorie intake to something like 800 calories per day. A one-meal-a-day intermittent fasting program will naturally limit calories consumed, but the reality is that there is no official limit of calorie intake. You can eat until you are satisfied during your 60-minute time window. A reduced-calorie diet will slow the metabolism, but that isn't the goal of intermittent fasting.

Calorie reduction not only slows the aging process; it has shown that limiting calorie intake by around 15% for an extended period lowers the risk of contracting many chronic "Western" diseases, including cancer, heart disease, Alzheimer's disease, and dementia. It is believed that these benefits stem from a slower metabolism, which results from being in a chronic state of consuming reduced calories. When the metabolism slows, there is less production of damaging free radicals.

Calorie reduction carried out over an extended period obviously leads to weight loss. As a result, many of the benefits attributed to radical calorie restrictive diets may be due to the simple fact that people who follow it are avoiding the problems that follow from being overweight and obese. However, there are far better ways to get fit and maintain a healthy weight, such as following a keto or paleo diet.

Something people who promote calorie restricted diets miss is that when you consume food, you are going to be replenishing glycogen in your liver and blood sugars are going to rise. Typically, calorie restricted diets are advised without any regard to food content. If you are consuming carbohydrates on a calorie restricted diet, then you are going to be utilizing blood sugar for energy. Weight loss will happen due to calorie deprivation, but you will not get the benefits that you will from outright fasting or from following a keto or low-carb diet, such as Atkins.

There are four ways that medical professionals measure calorie burning. The first way is called the *basal metabolic rate* or BMR. This is the rate at which calories are burned in order to maintain vital bodily functions. It is the minimal number of calories that your body needs to burn to keep the brain functioning, maintain heart rate, and keep you breathing. Put another way, BMR is the minimum necessary to get oxygen, pump blood, and stay conscious.

Two other ways that calories are burned are called *thermic effects*. Simply moving around causes the burning of calories, whether you are getting up to move from one chair to another or engaging in exercise. That type of calorie burning is called the thermic effect of exercise—that is calories burned while engaging in physical activity.

Related to this is "NEAT", which is a measure of calories burned in incidental movements, such as twiddling your thumbs. Nobody ever sits completely still, and if you watch a room full of high school students sitting at desks, you will notice that they are constantly fidgeting. This is called non-exercise activity thermogenesis—calories burned from fidgeting or moving around without getting up and utilizing your large muscle groups. For the most part, this type of activity occurs on a subconscious level, and younger people will burn more calories this way than older people who have "slowed down".

Another basic way you burn calories is by eating. Digestion is an active process, so it is going to burn off some calories. In fact, you burn up to 10% of the calories you consume by simply digesting a meal. This is called the thermal effect of food.

In summary, a calorie-restricted diet is more akin to entering a starvation state than it is to intermittent fasting. So-called starvation mode is a state the body enters when it feels it needs to conserve energy in response to a food-deprived state that can lead to the loss of life. If there is less energy coming into the body, then it attempts to maintain a balance by reducing energy expenditure, i.e., by slowing down the metabolism. The body will attempt to fight back, and in the short term will increase the sensation of hunger in order to motivate you to seek out and consume some calories.

Calorie restriction causes the levels of four hormones in your body to decrease. The first of these is the thyroid hormone. This hormone is important for maintaining the basal metabolic rate. Higher levels of the thyroid hormone will result in more oxygen consumption and energy utilization and lead to the production of more body heat. Deficiencies in the thyroid hormone are not normal and are treated by medical professionals for reasons outside the scope of this book; however, one thing to note is that people with lower levels of the thyroid hormone can have slightly lower body temperatures. Following a reduced-calorie diet can cause levels of the thyroid hormone to drop.

A reduced-calorie diet can also cause levels of a hormone called leptin to drop. Leptin is made by fat cells and acts inside your brain in a region called the hypothalamus. Leptin tends to inhibit hunger, so a drop in leptin levels can increase the sensation of hunger. You can see from this that a drop in leptin levels is part of the body's response of trying to get you to eat when it is faced with a reduced intake of calories.

Finally, when following a reduced-calorie diet, you will see a reduction in levels of the hormone norepinephrine. You can think of this hormone as a "fight or flight" hormone— in other words, it gets the body ready for taking action.

Seeing how the hormones impacted by a reduced-calorie diet act on the body, you can understand that someone following a constant reduced-calorie diet will be basically operating in a slowed down and semi-lethargic state. All dieting, of course, involves some level of calorie reduction. However, the levels of calorie consumption in the course of everyday life in modern societies involve the consumption of far more calories than we need. Second, a diet like keto naturally restricts calories without entering a starvation state. When you follow a diet like keto, you eat what your body needs but you are not entering a state of starvation like that advocated by practitioners of a calorie-restricted diet, and so you won't end up in a slowed down semi-deprived state.

One side effect of a strictly reduced-calorie diet—and that many people are put off by—is that it inevitably means a reduction of muscle mass. When the body faces continual deprivation in calories that are so low that they are near the level of actual starvation, the body will begin burning its own protein, which means it is going to burn your muscle mass. This causes further weight loss and slows the metabolism even more—since muscle tissue burns more energy over a given time frame than other tissues. If you think of the person following one of these extreme reduced-calorie diets as a sickly looking thin college professor with gray hair, a beard, and glasses, you are not far off the mark. However, when you are following a one-meal-a-day diet, you can avoid the problem of consuming your muscle mass by eating plenty of protein during your meal. Remember that protein intake is vital for the body to continue functioning, and it has to get protein from somewhere. In the absence of adequate protein intake, the body will break down muscle mass because the normal bodily processes that require proteins must continue in order to stay alive.

Those people who are utilizing the power of intermittent fasting are looking to achieve the health benefits of fasting without entering a starvation state, so looking to reduce calorie burning and slow the metabolism massively is not on the list of things to achieve. In fact, many people who are using intermittent fasting as a tool are looking to have a higher metabolism rather than entering a slowed down, restricted metabolism state of near starvation. Voluntarily restricting calories to a near-starvation level to increase lifespan actually sounds like a bad tradeoff. Why would you want an extended lifespan if you are a thin, slowed down shell of a person? It turns out that by using intermittent fasting, we can get many of the benefits of a reduced-calorie diet but without the downsides.

With weight loss comes some reduction of calorie expenditure. When you have less body tissue, you are simply burning fewer calories. Someone who weighs 200 pounds will burn more calories than someone who weighs 150 pounds by merely going through the days' activities and existing. Of course, you will get a headache if you try and figure out how many calories you're burning, and that is a detail you don't need to concern yourself with anyway. The only rule to be aware of is that it takes a deficit of 3,500 calories to burn off a pound of fat—or put another way, a pound of body fat stores 3,500 calories.

One-Meal-A-Day Intermittent Fasting isn't about deprivation

The purpose of the above discussion isn't to dissuade you from following a program of intermittent fasting; it should do the opposite. The effects of a chronically reduced-calorie diet of 800-1,000 calories per day (1,000 calories being the upper limit for men) are akin to being in a starvation state. If calories were restricted to smaller amounts, death would be the result, which is why the body attempts to fight against this state by encouraging hunger, consuming muscle mass, and slowing down the body's functions so that it can work more efficiently and consume fewer calories.

However, with intermittent fasting, some of our goals are the opposite of the things that result from following a severely calorie-restricted diet. Indeed, many people using intermittent fasting want to heighten, not reduce, their metabolism. People that follow a reduced-calorie diet are forced to take vitamin supplements. This is in contrast to a one-meal-a-day diet (although you can take supplements if you want). The most important thing to note is that while you are following a one-meal-a-day intermittent fasting diet, *you are not going to deprive your body of the vital nutrients it needs.* It is very easy to get adequate amounts of protein, vitamins, and minerals by eating just one meal a day. If you are following the keto diet, during your one meal per day, you will get all the fat that you need to burn for energy.

Summarizing, when following a one-meal-a-day diet:

- Each day, you let 23 hours pass until the next meal.

• You will not be counting calories. During the 60-minute eating window, you will eat until you are satisfied. Following a one-meal-a-day diet is not about trying to eat below a certain calorie level. If you get reduced-calorie consumption as a result and this helps with your weight loss goals, then this will be a benefit rather than a problem.

• You should eat enough protein to satisfy the needs of the body's basic functioning. Loss of muscle mass on a one-meal-a-day diet plan is not a goal; it's something that you should strive to avoid.

• A one-meal-a-day intermittent fasting plan does not involve any other deficiencies in nutrients—you should make sure that you get all the vitamins and minerals you need during your meal and by consuming bone broth.

How it works

A one-meal-a-day intermittent fasting plan does not involve any restrictions on calories. While generally speaking the program can be followed every single day, you can tailor it to your personal preferences. Just remember that if you don't use it every single day, you won't maximize the benefits; however, that does not mean you won't benefit at all. On the contrary, you can do it even just once a week and still get some of the benefits.

The number one goal of a one-meal-a-day intermittent fasting plan is to ensure that the body remains in a fat-burning mode and you reap some of the benefits from autophagy. This type of plan will work best with a low-carb diet. Keto is the perfect fit for an intermittent fasting plan because you are going to be in ketosis already and you won't be consuming any foods that knock you out of it and promote the replenishment of your glycogen stores. However, other methods of low-carb dieting can promote the same types of benefits. Before we get to those, let's take a look at the claims of keto dieters that you can't consume much protein on the diet without going out of ketosis.

Is too much protein a concern?

Ketogenic dieters emphasize that you should consume daily protein amounts that range between 0.5 g/lb to 0.9 g/lb where we are talking about grams of protein per pound of body mass. The claim is that excess protein will prevent you from entering ketosis. It turns out that this is not strictly true.

Your body needs protein for many functions. To implement many chemical processes, the body uses molecules called enzymes. An enzyme is what is called a catalyst—what this means is that a given chemical reaction will proceed at a faster and stronger rate in the presence of the enzyme as compared to the absence of the enzyme. Without enzymes in the body, many chemical reactions that are necessary for life would occur too slowly, produce far too few results, or not even happen at all. In short, enzymes are necessary for complex life to exist. And as it turns out, enzymes are made of protein.

You also need protein to build muscle mass and cut fat. So, if you are seeking a leaner, more muscled, and toned body, getting adequate protein is essential.

Protein is also required for healthy skin and nails, and proper brain functioning. The good news is that if you on a normal diet (that is not purposefully severely calorie restricted) the chances are that you are going to get more than enough adequate protein. However, those eating at the lower limit of the recommendations for a keto diet can run into some problems, and those will be mostly limited to reduced muscle mass. The body is going to utilize protein where it is needed first, so making enzymes and keeping your brain and heart muscles healthy is going to take priority over bigger biceps.

The worry that keto dieters have over protein is related to a process known as *gluconeogenesis*. This is a process that occurs in periods of carbohydrate deprivation. In short, the liver can make glucose out of protein. If carbohydrate intake is severely restricted, then it will make some glucose out of any excess protein that is consumed. The result of this will be knocking the body out of ketosis due to rising blood sugar levels—or so goes the belief of keto dieters.

However, is this really true? The Atkins diet calls this into question. This diet, formulated in the late 1960s and early 1970s, was the first diet that promoted being in ketosis to lose weight, and which hit the mainstream. The Atkins diet encourages liberal consumption of fat but makes no claims about daily macro consumption, other than restrictions on carbohydrate intake. In the induction phase of Atkins, dieters are required to restrict daily carbohydrate intake to twenty grams of net carbs per day or less.

Aside: To calculate the net carbs of any food, take the total carbohydrates, and subtract the dietary fiber. The leftover is net carbs, which are carbs that your body can burn for energy and hence raise your blood sugar.

As a practical matter, Atkins dieters who follow these guidelines without any worry as to total protein intake lose large amounts of weight—in comparable amounts to those experienced by keto dieters. Some Atkins dieters may be limiting protein intake to levels promoted by keto dieters without really thinking about it, but the scientific research points to the idea that limiting protein levels isn't necessary for promoting ketosis—provided that you are getting significant fat in your diet.

Where people mess up when it comes to ketosis, protein, and blood sugar is by consuming protein that is too lean without making up for the fat elsewhere.

People also make mistakes by consuming what is known in the diet industry as "hidden carbs". Hidden carbs are all around us; they might be in a barbecue rub, sauces, and condiments. There are even hidden carbs in high-fat products like heavy cream. Carbs are minimal in heavy cream, but if you use a lot of it throughout the day, you may be getting more carbs in your diet than you think. About 3% of the calories in heavy cream come from carbohydrates. If you consume about eight tablespoons, you are getting 3.3 grams of carbs. It is true—that isn't much—but if you are trying to limit your total daily consumption of carbs to twenty grams, then it adds up and can tip you over. So, if you are following a low-carb diet, make sure that the amounts of carbohydrates that you think you are getting are really an accurate count.

Another source of hidden carbs is organ meats. After all, how many times have you heard about glycogen in the liver? Remember that glycogen is a form of starch. So if you are eating chicken liver, you're getting some starch in the diet. Some low-carb dieters neglect to count carbs from these sources.

The key takeaway message is that protein consumption in conjunction with fat will not kick you out of ketosis. The only time protein consumption will be a worry is if you eat lean meat together with other low-fat food items. To avoid this kind of problem, eat your meat with the fat it naturally contains. That means eat steak with the fat on it and poultry and fish with the skin. If you do make a dish with a low-fat or lean meat item like skinless chicken breasts, use a butter-based sauce and include a healthy serving of olive oil on your veggies, or add in a high-fat food item like avocados.

And what about gluconeogenesis? The reality is that it's a completely natural process, and you can't shut it off. But it's not a danger to knocking you out of ketosis. In fact, your body must maintain a minimal amount of blood sugar.

Not all tissues can run on ketones

If you are following the keto diet—and no doubt you have at least studied it, or you wouldn't be interested in intermittent fasting—then you have probably heard of all the wonders the keto diet does for the brain. After all, the keto diet was first used to treat children who had epilepsy. The scientific basis of this is not in dispute by anyone, so it is clear that ketones do affect the brain and positively.

However, something keto dieters don't tell you is the brain cannot function entirely on ketones. In fact, ketones can only supply the brain with about 70% of its total energy needs. So, for your brain to stay healthy and function at optimal levels, it needs some glucose.

Second, other cells in the body must be fueled with glucose. They are a minority, but they are also important. For example, red blood cells need glucose. Obviously, without red blood cells, your body would not function for very long. Other cells that need glucose are certain types of kidney cells and cells in the testicles.

Glycogen isn't just for the liver

Discussions of intermittent fasting and ketogenic diets often talk about glycogen. The problem with these discussions is that they only focus on glycogen in the liver. It is true that if your liver is stocked up on glycogen when you adopt a ketogenic lifestyle or engage in intermittent fasting, your body will continue running on blood sugar until the liver's glycogen stores have been burned off.

However, that isn't the only place where you have glycogen in your body. Large stores of glycogen are also found in your muscle cells. Unless you are not physically active, you're going to need to replenish the glycogen in your muscles. Your muscles rely on that glycogen to act and recover from workouts.

Hypoglycemia

Hypoglycemia is a condition that results when blood sugar levels drop below a minimum amount, <70 mg/dL. If left untreated, it can be very serious, resulting in a coma. Most people that get hypoglycemia have diabetes, and the treatment involves getting a lot of blood sugar in their system through the consumption of sugar either directly or through high sugar foods like fruit juice. The first symptoms of hypoglycemia are anxiety, irritability, extreme hunger, and shakiness. As it progresses, the patient can develop heart arrhythmias, tingling around the mouth, visual disturbances, and mental confusion. This can progress into seizures, and if not treated, a coma and death. True hypoglycemia is not typically a concern for people who do not have diabetes.

The role of gluconeogenesis

The body utilizes gluconeogenesis to deal with and prevent the problems described above. In other words, the body utilizes gluconeogenesis in the absence of a large intake of carbohydrates when in ketosis to ensure that blood sugar levels are adequate to:

- Keep the brain 100% fueled.
- Make sure red blood cells, kidney cells, and other cells that can't utilize ketosis have energy.
- Prevent hypoglycemia.

So, the reality is that your body is going to be engaging in some level of gluconeogenesis no matter what you do—because the body cannot function 100% on ketosis or continue if blood sugar levels drop in the hypoglycemic range.

So now you know that you need some level of gluconeogenesis. However, the most important fact to know is that your body does not engage in gluconeogenesis to excess. So eating a relatively large amount of protein by itself is not going to kick you out of ketosis.

There are two important points. One is that you will get more than enough protein if you are eating around a gram per pound of body weight each day. That will keep you from having muscle loss, and be adequate for weight training for most people. The second is that it is hard to go beyond that. If you weigh 180 pounds, one gram per pound is 180 grams. That is a lot of protein—consider how a pound of 70% lean hamburger contains just 65 grams of protein (however, for 93% lean ground beef, the figure is about 96 grams of protein).

In short, you shouldn't spend your time obsessing too much on protein consumption unless you are a bodybuilder—in which case you will want to get more protein, not less. Just don't worry about it knocking you out of ketosis.

Of course, the important thing with dieting is to personalize your lifestyle plan. So the best thing to do is get a ketosis meter and find out how the consumption of different foods and amounts of protein impact your body over several days.

The best types of diets for intermittent fasting

With intermittent fasting, one of the primary goals is to promote the following changes:

- Reduction of insulin levels.
- Depletion of glycogen stores in the liver.
- Increase glucagon levels.
- Promote fat burning—in particular, our stores of body fat.

With that in mind, the best approach to intermittent fasting is to consume a daily meal that is congruent to meeting those goals. We should note that intermittent fasting, especially when we are talking about a one-meal-a-day program where we have gotten to the maximum length of a fasting period that we can without fasting for more than one entire day, is compatible with nearly any kind of diet. It won't be compatible with spending your hour of food consumption eating high fructose corn syrup and junk food—because that kind of food gets burned off very quickly and would cause your blood sugars to plummet after a large spike. As a result, you would find yourself quickly getting hungry and have major difficulties in pursuing 23 hours of food deprivation.

Hence, the kind of meals that are compatible with a one-meal-a-day intermittent fasting plan are those that involve the consumption of natural, wholesome foods. You can consume carbohydrates if desired; however, you should note that if you consume carbohydrates in a manner that is inconsistent with a low-carb diet, your liver is going to replenish its glycogen stores. That means every day that you are going into the fasting state you're basically fighting the same battle. The first twelve hours of your fast, at a minimum, are going to be spent burning off the glycogen. This will act to limit the amount of time your body spends in burning off body fat for energy.

A paleo diet is better than a standard American diet when it comes to intermittent fasting. Strictly speaking, paleo diets do not place upper limits on carbohydrate consumption. They allow you to consume natural food items like sweet potatoes and strawberries that may consume significant amounts of sugars, and some paleo dieters eat fruit like oranges and apples as well. However, if you are following a paleo diet closely, you're more likely to limit yourself to berries and root vegetables like turnips. The result is that, compared to a standard American diet, you are going to be eating fewer carbs in absolute terms and as an overall fraction of your diet. Many paleo dieters also work to limit their overall carbohydrate consumption.

Any low-carb diet that limits total daily consumption of carbohydrates to 60 grams or less per day will be compatible with intermittent fasting. However, remember that if you are following paleo or a mildly low-carb eating plan, there is still going to be at least some replenishment of glycogen in the liver. Any amount of glycogen in the liver is going to slow down the process of entering a truly fasted state. Moreover, if you are following a limited-carbohydrate diet and are in a state of mild ketosis, you might find yourself spending some time out of ketosis as the body increases blood sugar by burning through the glycogen stores in the liver.

A diet that limits daily carbohydrate consumption to twenty grams of carbs per day or less will be the diet that is best suited to incorporating intermittent fasting. This is the case whether or not you are following keto or some other low-carb diet like Atkins or South Beach. However, a diet that incorporates the consumption of high amounts of fat is going to work best.

By consuming high amounts of fat, your body will be in a state of ketosis by default and your liver is not going to be loaded up on glycogen. As a result, when you engage in intermittent fasting, you are going to be in a fasted state far quicker than you would be if you were consuming higher amounts of carbohydrates.

Tips on Eating with One-Meal-A-Day Fasting

The first thing to realize with one meal per day intermittent fasting is that you need to consume adequate amounts of calories. The goal is not only to reap the benefits of fasting but to heighten the metabolism as well, and burn off lots of body fat. You don't want the body to get into a state where it "believes" starvation is beginning and so it needs to conserve energy. You can do this by making sure you are getting a proper, balanced diet:

- Ensure that your meal provides adequate protein needs for your body size and type, and activity levels. If you engage in strength training, you may need a little more extra protein.
- Make sure you consume enough fat. You don't want to leave your meal without being satiated.
- Pay attention to your vitamins and minerals. The point of intermittent fasting is to get the benefits of fasting but without the downsides of nutrient depletion. This means, in particular, getting proper amounts of sodium, potassium, magnesium, and calcium. These minerals are vital for the proper functioning of your digestive system, heart muscle (and heart rhythms), and avoiding problems like muscle cramping. You can supplement with bone broth if you feel you are not getting enough, but be sure to read labels to know what you're actually getting with bone broth.
- Keep your meal diverse. Since you're only getting one meal per day, it's important to avoid just eating meat. Make sure you get adequate intake of vegetables and fruits. For a low-carb dieter, fruits come in the form of avocados, coconut, and olives. A healthy intake of leafy green vegetables and coniferous vegetables can help you maintain health with a diverse diet that includes spinach, kale, and

broccoli. You'll also be sure to check your fiber intake to maintain proper digestion. Fiber can come in the form of nuts, avocados, and leafy green vegetables.

• Watch your calcium. To make sure you aren't becoming calcium deficient, which can lead to many problems that don't just include osteoporosis, you want to get some natural calcium in your diet. If drinking whole milk fits within your carbohydrate limits, you can do that, but eating cheese is a good way to get calcium without going over on carbs. Be sure to eat full-fat cheese and avoid low-fat varieties.

• Eat until satisfied. The goal with your one meal isn't to gorge yourself; you want to eat until you're satiated and have the proper level of nutrients for the day. This way, you can reduce overall daily caloric intake, which helps with weight loss but do it in a way that doesn't put the body in starvation mode and hence reduce your metabolism.

Carnivore Dieting and One-Meal-A-Day Intermittent Fasting

The carnivore diet is one diet that is very compatible with this type of fasting. In fact, many practitioners of the carnivore diet already eat this way without consciously thinking about it. They will sit down for their big porterhouse steak and be completely satisfied, and not need to eat for the rest of the day. The requirements for a carnivore diet are different from those with a keto or Atkins diet, so the focus here won't be eating to get fiber and vegetables; you want to focus instead solely on eating until you feel you have had enough. While a carnivore diet is beyond the scope of this book, in general, you can eat any animal products that you deem fit. Some carnivore dieters pursue "zero-carb" dieting, while others allow themselves to consume organ meats and some dairy products.

Liquids throughout the day

A one meal per day intermittent fasting program is not a dry fast. As a result, you are advised to consume copious amounts of water throughout the day, as needed. Later, you will learn more about how one mistake people new to an intermittent fasting program make is not getting enough water. In any detoxification procedure getting enough water is important to help flush out the body and maintain healthy digestion. As you will see with autophagy, getting adequate amounts of water will turn out to be important.

A word of warning when it comes to consuming coffee and tea: While calories are zero or minimal with such beverages, remember that these are stimulants that are also diuretics. That means that they encourage your body to produce more urine, and when you are urinating more, it means that your body will get low on fluids. If you are drinking coffee or teas during the day, you will need to be sure to make up for it by drinking more water to make up for the deficit. It is important to stay properly hydrated while using intermittent fasting so that you maximize the possible benefits. Frequent urination also causes mineral depletion, so if you drink these types of drinks, watch your sodium, potassium, and magnesium.

You should also avoid artificial sweeteners while consuming these products. Strictly speaking, they claim to be low calorie or even zero calories, but they can trick the body into thinking it is getting calories. It's also turning out that claims of being zero calories or having no impact on blood sugar may be exaggerated. If you are going to use artificial sweeteners, you should restrict their use to periods during which you are not fasting—for a one meal per day intermittent fasting program that means using them during your 60-minute consumption window.

What about alcohol? You will probably want to avoid it on most fasting days. However, if you are going to consume it, do so in moderation and during the 60-minute consumption window because alcoholic beverages do contain calories. If you are following a keto or carnivore diet, you should stick to the types of alcoholic beverages that minimize carbohydrates. This includes most types of wine and hard liquors like brandy or vodka. An important note about alcohol is that like caffeinated beverages, alcoholic drinks act as diuretics, causing increased urination and hence fluid and mineral loss. So, if you do drink alcohol, be sure to drink extra water.

Finally, a word about bone broth to close the discussion about beverages: You can consume bone broth during a fast to help keep your sodium and other mineral levels up. However, be aware that bone broth, while having minimal calories, is not calorie free. Typically, a cup of bone broth will have 30 calories.

What Happens when the body enters the fasting state?

For the moment, do not worry about whether or not you are following a ketogenic diet, so you can learn how the body operates when you fast. When you stop consuming food, the body will immediately burn through its available supply of carbohydrates, whether this is the food you have just consumed or carbs in your liver. You can understand how this works better by considering an analogy—money. Carbohydrates are like "easy money", or put another way, cash on hand. It is easy for the body to burn carbs, just like it's easy for you to spend cash. What is not so easy for you to spend? Assets that are not "liquid"—as they say in financial lingo. This means assets that cannot be quickly turned into cash. For example, you might own some stocks, a 401k, or an IRA. If you wanted to, with a bit of pain, you could get the cash out from those assets. But it takes a little work and time. However, if you have a significant amount of money invested in stocks and other assets of that type, you can use it to live off of over a long period, which is what many people do in retirement.

Fat is kind of like the "stocks" of nutrition. It is less easily spent on energy than sugar, but it can power the body over the long term. Over the first day of fasting, carbohydrates are very quickly burned off. Proteins, which are only utilized for a relatively small amount of daily energy, peak a bit at the beginning of a fasting period, but not by much. The utilization of proteins quickly drops off and slowly but steadily declines as time goes on. However, protein utilization doesn't drop off completely and stays fairly constant. Carbohydrate utilization drops off far more rapidly and to lower levels.

When you enter into a period of fasting, fat utilization quickly ramps up. Most of the *increase* in fat utilization for energy will happen within the first hours and certainly within the first day of fasting. It will rise to a peak after a few days, and taper off a little with time. Of course, most people are only looking at fasting for, at most, a day, so that eventual dropping off of energy production by burning fat isn't a concern.

As long as the body doesn't enter starvation mode, the protein will not be consumed very much, and the body will conserve protein as much as possible, even in a fasting state when you are not consuming any external protein sources.

In the initial phases of fasting, the body will attempt to continue burning sugar, and that is what the glycogen stores are for in the liver. Remember that sugar is easy money. You can think of the cash you usually have in your wallet that you can spend immediately as blood sugar that comes from carbohydrates consumed while eating. Money in your piggy bank or bank account that you can quickly access with an ATM is like glycogen stored in the liver.

When that money runs out, you are going to have to get energy from somewhere else. If you didn't have any money in a bank account but had a large stock portfolio, you would have to cash some of it out. Analogously, if you've already depleted the glycogen in your liver, then your body will more easily transition to burning its body fat for energy. You can either go through a 12-hour or so period of burning off the glycogen in your liver every time you fast, or you can get a head start by following a low carbohydrate high-fat diet. That way, you will be able to utilize most of those twelve hours burning your body fat.

How Does Fasting Prevent or Even Reverse Diabetes?

Many people come to intermittent fasting hoping that they can find a way to get faster fat loss—and the truth is fasting can do that. However, that is not the only health benefit that you can get from following an intermittent fasting program. One of the most important benefits of fasting comes from its ability to reset the metabolic system and reduce the risks of diabetes. In fact, even if you have diabetes, in some cases, diabetes can be eliminated by fasting, or at least its severity can be curtailed.

Losing weight has long been recognized as an important way to prevent the development of diabetes, especially among people who are already having blood sugar and other metabolic problems and have been diagnosed as "pre-diabetic". Moreover, people with diabetes can see their health improve if they are overweight, and they lose weight in order to achieve healthy weight levels. For these reasons alone, fasting can help prevent and reverse diabetes.

However, the main reasons intermittent fasting is beneficial are those that happen below the surface, not available to the "naked eye". Intermittent fasting causes many biochemical changes inside the body that make diabetes less likely, or that can help reverse it if you already have diabetes.

One way it does this is by stopping blood sugar spikes. People who are pre-diabetic or diabetic experience large blood sugar spikes after consuming a meal that contains significant levels of carbohydrates. As discussed earlier, blood sugar spikes damage the small capillaries and blood vessels in the body, and over time, this can lead to organ damage and heart disease. However, blood sugar spikes in and of themselves are not diabetes, but rather a symptom of diabetes.

Next are blood sugar levels themselves, on an average basis. Your average blood sugar level can be tracked for the past 90 days by measuring your A1C level. Diabetics and pre-diabetics have higher A1C levels because their blood sugars are already high. Studies have proven that people with diabetes who engage in intermittent fasting have lower A1C levels when compared to diabetics who are not engaging in fasting.

One problem that some studies have shown is that people with diabetes who fast suffer from hypoglycemic episodes. However, this stems from two problems. The first is that studies have shown this involves diabetics who are using intermittent fasting but eating whatever they want on non-fasting days. So, in other words, many of the study participants were consuming large amounts of carbohydrates while eating. You can see why this would lead to a problem with low blood sugars—when you suddenly pull the sugar fuel away, the body cannot adjust, and low blood sugars are the result.

This situation is made worse by the fact that diagnosed diabetics are on one or more medications that can cause blood sugars to drop. These include metformin and insulin, plus a large number of newer and very potent drugs. Medical professionals attempt to adjust the medications during studies of people with diabetes who are on fasting programs; however, this is not always achievable in the right amounts, and some patients will experience hypoglycemic episodes. Part of this reflects the paradigm that so many people are caught up in—that is, it is normal to eat large amounts of carb-laden foods day in and day out. With that brainwashing myth infecting so many in the medical community, it is not surprising that they would advise their patients to eat high-carb diets (filled with fruits and "whole grains") and then face low blood sugars when the medications are continued, but the food sources are withdrawn. These problems can be minimized if not eliminated by getting rid of the real problem—

which is carbohydrates in the diet in the first place. If you are never eating carbohydrates, then you don't need nearly as much insulin and won't have blood sugar spikes or crashes. Of course, any person with diabetes should engage in fasting only under the advice and consent of their doctor.

Insulin levels are one problem that people who are prone to diabetes suffer from. Specifically, a pre-diabetic will have high insulin levels coupled with reduced insulin sensitivity, or insulin resistance. Intermittent fasting is a potent weapon for anyone who is pre-diabetic but has yet to be put on medications. In that situation, the first thing that fasting is going to do is cause an overall reduction in blood levels of insulin. Over time, with reduced amounts of insulin in the environment, cells will begin to get their insulin sensitivity back. In short, a metabolic reset takes place, leaving the body in a healthier state overall.

You don't have to be pre-diabetic or diabetic to benefit from these changes. In fact, even if you aren't diagnosed as pre-diabetic, if you are overweight, you are probably heading in that direction. In that case, you can start to benefit now by incorporating intermittent fasting to reset your insulin system and lose weight before it really starts to become a problem. If you are only mildly overweight, you can nip it in the bud even earlier.

Autophagy Explained

So, you have seen that a one-meal-a-day intermittent fasting program will lead to weight loss and help heal the insulin hormonal system. While that is beneficial enough, one of the reasons so many people are incorporating intermittent fasting into their lifestyle is that it also promotes a cleansing process called *autophagy*. In short, autophagy means to eat oneself. While that concept sounds crazy, as we will see, there are very good reasons for it.

It is a fact of life that, with time, all things become worn out and break down. This happens no matter how much effort is put into keeping things up. Sure, you can keep up an old car, but it will take a lot of time, money, and energy. You can repaint the car now and then, and spend a large amount of money on maintenance and upkeep. Parts will have to be routinely replaced, and you may even have to replace the transmission or the engine. New tires are in order fairly frequently, and brakes will have to be serviced. You can also prolong the life of the car by not using it very much.

Of course, in your body, you don't have the option of not using your cells. And the ways of the world being what they are, your cells wear down just like old cars do. In the process, they become less efficient and so require more energy to maintain the same level of function. They also become worn out on the inside, as internal parts (called "organelles" by scientists) get worn out as well. Debris from dead or worn out parts accumulates inside the cell, making efficiency a problem.

If you are suffering through an old car that continually breaks down, eventually you're going to give up on it and replace it with a new car that works better.

You would like the same thing to happen within the body. One way this procedure occurs is in the process of cell birth; for example, your bone marrow is constantly making new blood cells. Another process called apoptosis occurs where cells die when programmed to do so. That procedure ensures that cells that are too old and causing problems just sitting around are not allowed to exist.

Before a car is completely worn out, you can replace parts to keep it on the road for a prolonged period. For example, when your tires or brakes are worn out, you don't rush to the dealership to trade it in. Most of the car is functioning fine, so you are more likely simply to get new tires and brakes. Cells work the same way. The cell itself might be fine, but some of its internal parts or organelles may be worn out and turned into waste products. One thing to do to keep the cell functioning properly, and hence to extend its life in the same way you would with a good car that just needs new brakes, is to clean out the dead and useless debris from inside the cell. Just like dysfunctional brakes, peeling paint and old filters are a sign that a car is getting older, dysfunctional organelles and the accumulation of old, battered cells in the body are one major sign of aging.

There are several types of cells in your body whose job it is to destroy things. Often, the things these cells destroy are outside intruders you don't want like invading bacteria or viruses. So we see that these cells are part of the immune system. One type of cell that fits this role is lysosomes. It was by studying lysosomes that scientists were able to connect them to the processes that take place in the body during fasting.

By studying rats, scientists found that the number of lysosomes in the liver increased when the rats were given injections of glucagon. Remember from the first chapter that glucagon is a hormone that acts in concert with but in opposite ways to insulin. Think of insulin as the storage hormone—it promotes storage of starches in the liver, cells to use blood sugar, and excess blood sugar to be stored away as fat. Glucagon is the storage usage hormone, so it promotes the body to use up whatever glycogen is stored in the liver and then to use up body fat for energy. So what the researchers really found was that glucagon activates cells that engage in autophagy.

Of course, one way to promote the levels of glucagon in your system is by intermittent fasting.

When you were a kid, you might have played on a seesaw. When one kid goes up, the other goes down and vice versa. The relationship between insulin and glucagon is like that. Insulin goes up in response to the consumption of food (mostly carbohydrates). When insulin goes up, glucagon levels go down—vice versa, in times of food deprivation, insulin levels drop while levels of glucagon go up. It can be no other way; if this type of relationship didn't exist, then the body would be battling with itself since insulin and glucagon act in nearly opposite ways.

So, during fasting, glucagon levels go up. And as indicated from the original rat study, and this has been borne many times since, when glucagon levels go up, autophagy is stimulated within the body's tissues. As a result, old cellular debris (parts no longer functioning) and old cells are marked for destruction. The immune system then goes to work, eliminating this material from your body. Think of it like replacing the brakes and tires on the car that is starting to get older; it slows down the aging process and gives your body a rejuvenated sense of life.

The process of autophagy is believed to continue in the body for about two days after it is initiated during fasting. Eating will actually turn off the process of autophagy. This is why longer periods of fasting are more beneficial for health than short periods, such as 16:8 fasting. If you are using 16:8 fasting, if you start autophagy at all, it won't last very long.

In fact, consuming any level of calories will turn off the process of autophagy. So a reduced-calorie diet that many are advocating—or "fasting" but allowing the consumption of a small number of calories during the day (usually 500-800)—will turn off autophagy or prevent it from being initiated. There is only one way to trigger the process, and that is to fast for a long enough period. For that reason, you should avoid consuming bone broth during your fasting time. If you are following a one meal per day intermittent fasting plan, it shouldn't be an issue. During your 60-minute eating window, you can consume as much bone broth as you want.

How Long to Fast to Trigger Autophagy

Autophagy doesn't start the instant you begin fasting; it begins when the liver's store of glycogen is depleted. So you have to fast between twelve-sixteen hours to trigger the process of autophagy. Here again, we see the benefits of following a ketogenic or low-carb diet. If you are following that type of diet, then the glycogen stores in the liver are at a lower level than they will be for someone who is consuming carbohydrates. As a result, when you engage in intermittent fasting, you will be able to start the process of autophagy much faster.

The Benefits of Autophagy

Autophagy is like a "spring cleaning" that clears out all the junk in your house. However, it has many benefits that aren't related to losing weight, so fasting can be beneficial even for people who are maintaining normal weight levels.

Slowing the Aging Process

By cleaning out all the junk, whether it is old broken down cells or worn out cell parts, the body slows down the aging process. Fasting also promotes human growth hormone, which helps promote the birth of new cells and the construction of new parts, in essence, rebuilding anew in place. This helps the body remain youthful and rejuvenated. You can think of autophagy as a natural "fountain of youth"—something that people have dreamed about for centuries but have never been able to grasp.

Reduced Risk of Alzheimer's

Some diseases are characterized by if not caused by junk laying around. Old sticky proteins can prevent the normal functioning of your cells, and this is true when it comes to Alzheimer's disease. When you suffer from this disease, old dysfunctional proteins pile up in the brain. Almost everyone probably has this happen to one degree or another, and so autophagy helping clean things up is very beneficial and can reduce the risk of contracting this dreadful disease.

Mental Clarity and Revitalizing the Nervous System

Alzheimer's isn't the only condition that can benefit from autophagy. In fact, the nervous system, whether you have the proteins associated with Alzheimer's accumulating in your brain or not, will benefit from autophagy. Autophagy has been shown to increase mental clarity, enhance nervous system function, and encourage neuroplasticity, which is the process by which the brain rewires itself when exposed to new information. In other words, the brain becomes better at learning and memory as a result of autophagy "cleaning house".

Reduced Risk of Cancer

Since fasting triggers autophagy, which is basically immune cells going around and cleaning out unwanted junk and old cells, it also may trigger the cleaning up of cancer cells in the very earliest stages of development.

Reversing Damage to Healthy Tissues and Organs

The process of being alive is simply dangerous, due to the production of free radicals in addition to the usual wear and tear. Autophagy can help combat this and revitalize organs and tissues by clearing out old, ineffective parts.

Improved Regulation of Mitochondria

Mitochondria are the energy powerhouses of the cell, where much of the energy production and metabolism takes place. Like everything else, mitochondria are subject to oxidative stress and damage. Autophagy can help repair the damage and therefore keep mitochondria operating at full potential, supplying the vital energy needs of your cells.

Promoting Heart Health

Some studies have shown that autophagy may trigger the development of new heart cells, helping keep your heart stronger, young, and vital.

Myths Associated with One-Meal-A-Day Fasting

There are many myths associated with fasting, but most of these arise out of common misperceptions of what fasting is all about. In particular, many medical professionals seem steeped in old ways of viewing things that aren't accurate and associated with the belief that you should be consuming a diet that derives at least 50% of its calories from carbohydrates.

Let's take a look at some of the myths:

One-Meal-A-Day Intermittent Fasting is starvation

We have seen a difference between starvation and fasting. To begin with, starvation has no end point—perhaps rescue or death? Secondly, starvation is involuntary.

In contrast, one meal per day intermittent fasting is voluntary and has an endpoint. The fasting period ends every single day when you decide to eat, which is at the 23-hour mark from your previous meal.

Second, while starvation involves the brutal deprivation of nutrients, as well as macros like protein, one meal per day intermittent fasting does the opposite. You are keeping your body very well fed on a one meal per day intermittent fasting program. You are simply compressing the period during which you consume all the nutrients that you need into a single hour.

One-Meal-A-Day Intermittent Fasting slows down the metabolism

This myth arises in part from the first myth. That is, people are brainwashed into equating fasting and starvation. When the body is in starvation mode, it will slow down its metabolism in response, attempting to conserve energy it thinks it will need in the future. After all, if you are truly starving, then you don't know when your next meal will come—if it comes at all. In contrast, on a one meal per day plan, you completely take in all of your nutritional components every single day. This ensures that your body will not slow down its metabolism. Although you are depriving your body of food intake for 23 hours, in the end, the body gets all the nutrients that it needs for the entire 24-hour period. So it is not going to slow down the metabolism, and many people actually experience a heightened metabolism while following a program of intermittent fasting.

One-Meal-A-Day Intermittent Fasting causes hypoglycemia

One meal per day intermittent fasting is not going to cause hypoglycemia in most people. This is because the body will be getting energy from stored body fat, after the glycogen stores in the liver have been run out. In fact, there are only a small group of people who are at risk of hypoglycemic incidents while doing intermittent fasting, and these are type 1 and type 2 diabetics. Type 1 diabetics are completely insulin dependent (meaning they can only get it through medications, and they have to regulate their usage of these medications carefully). Type 2 diabetics may also be dependent on insulin and taking one or more blood sugar controlling drugs. These drugs are, to a certain extent, a trap in that the patient must consume a certain level of carbohydrates to prevent them from becoming hypoglycemic. However, when it comes to hypoglycemic incidents, if they do happen with type 2 diabetics, it is because their medications have not been adjusted properly. This is the fault of the doctors or careless patients who did not seek out the advice of their doctor before fasting. If you have type 2 diabetes, be sure to closely work with your doctor while you are engaging in fasting.

If you do not have diabetes, or at least aren't pre-diabetic, a hypoglycemic incident is extremely unlikely. Not only will your body keep up blood glucose levels in adequate amounts through gluconeogenesis, but your body will quickly switch over to fat burning as well.

Fasting burns muscle mass

Fasting only burns muscle mass if you engage in prolonged fasting or fail to get proper nutrition when you are eating. We can quickly dispense with the first situation because, with one-meal-a-day fasting, you are never going to be lacking for nutrients. You can eat whatever you want and need during your 60-minute daily eating period. Certainly, during that period, you can and should get whatever protein is necessary. Second, this has been proven by scientific research on people who engage in intermittent fasting. Some studies have shown that the loss of body fat occurs at nearly twice the amount that total body weight is lost while engaging in intermittent fasting. Some weight will be lost due to water weight, so what this means is intermittent fasting almost entirely burns off body fat. A bit of lean body mass lost during fasting is connective tissue and skin. Some studies have explicitly shown that lean body mass, aka muscle tissue, is easily maintained during intermittent fasting. If this is a fear you have, calculate how much protein your body needs, and then make sure that you are getting that amount during your eating period each day. Suffering from the loss of muscle mass is very low risk since following the one meal per day fasting pattern means you're eating daily.

Reduced-calorie diets prove intermittent fasting isn't as beneficial as claimed

In fact, reduced-calorie diets prove absolutely nothing about intermittent fasting. We have seen that following a reduced-calorie diet has some limited benefits by increasing lifespan and slowing down the aging process. However, these benefits are complicated by the fact that reduced-caloric intake results in a slowed metabolism and does not promote the hormonal benefits of intermittent fasting. Remember that if you consume any foods, you are not going to activate autophagy, and you're also not going to see increases in growth hormones (in fact, quite the opposite). Reduced-calorie consumption will also not activate glucagon and keep insulin levels elevated, even though the degree to which they are elevated is lower than that seen with normal eating patterns. In short, reduced-calorie intake is not fasting, and so shouldn't be confused with fasting.

Intermittent fasting promotes overeating

Studies have shown this not to be the case. For example, people who follow a true fasting period of 24 hours or even 48 hours will consume a large number of calories on the first day that they return to eating food. However, research shows that when you average out the number of calories for the entire period, they consumed much fewer calories than they would have continuing to follow normal eating patterns. Secondly, the eating binge that follows when immediately going off a fast tends to be a one-time event.

In the case of a one-meal-a-day intermittent fasting program, since you are not going the entire day without eating, and you continue eating day in and day out, you are not going to find yourself engaging in binge behavior. That is only a risk—if at all—if you are going on an extended fast.

One-Meal-A-Day Intermittent Fasting Mistakes

While the principles are simple, mistakes can be made that can keep you from getting maximum health benefits from your intermittent fasting program. Let's look at some of the top mistakes beginners make when taking up fasting:

Not getting enough water

Getting enough water is important on two levels. For one, it is necessary to maintain a feeling of wellbeing and alertness when you are fasting. If you are experiencing low energy levels, consider drinking more water. However, water consumption is important in more ways than one! In any detox program, water consumption is important to help flush out the system. When you are going through autophagy, you're also going to need more water than you would under normal circumstances.

Cheating on the fast

Unfortunately, the advocates of the 5:2 diet promoted the idea that you can still eat and be considered fasting as long as the number of calories is limited. This is false. If you consume calories during the fasting period, then you are not fasting; instead, you are following a reduced-calorie diet. The most important aspect of this is that the consumption of any calories will turn off the process of autophagy, and it will also inhibit the activity of glucagon and growth hormone. The results will be that you see fewer benefits in terms of slowing down the aging process, weight loss, reduced blood pressure, and rejuvenation.

Binge eating

Overeating should not be a problem with one-meal-a-day intermittent fasting. However, some people give into binge eating. Since we are talking about a fasting program where you do eat during the day, even though it is only over one hour, if you binge eat, it is possible to end up consuming too many calories. If you are finding yourself not losing weight, despite strictly following an intermittent fasting program, take a look at how many calories you are consuming during your meal.

Eating too late at night

One of the first studies on intermittent fasting examined what happened if people avoided eating at night. One of the things discovered was that the more you let eating intrude on the time before going to sleep, the less ability you have to meet your weight loss goals. This is old advice that you may have even heard from your grandmother. With one-meal-a-day intermittent fasting, you should consider eating your meal as early as possible. You should be finished by eight p.m. at the latest, and earlier than that is certainly ideal.

Giving up too easily

The first few times you fast, you may find it difficult. You may experience some irritability, feelings of anxiety, and a focus on food and hunger. Those who are not ketosis adjusted may experience weakness. Some people find this enough reason to give up the idea of fasting. However, if you work through them instead, then you will find that each time you fast, you get better at it and find it more tolerable.

Thinking daily fasting is the only way

One thing about fasting is that any fasting program can be personalized. One-meal-a-day intermittent fasting is no different. If you want to do it daily, you can if you feel your body adjusts to it well. It is also possible to do it every other day, or just two-three days per week. You can even only do it one day per week and get some of the benefits. Rather than finding that doing it daily is something you don't care to do, and thus quitting, personalize your fasting program and find a frequency that works for you. You can also work it in with other types of fasting to maximize the benefits. For example, you can do 16:8 fasting three-five days a week, and then do one-meal-a-day fasting in between. There are no hard and fast rules here.

Drinking too much coffee and/or tea

Consuming beverages that contain caffeine can be a problem. No rule says you cannot consume these beverages; in fact, you most certainly can. The problem is that they will leave you in a state of dehydration and possibly mineral deficient. If you are the kind of person who cannot live with a certain amount of coffee or tea throughout the day, be sure to get extra water during fasting to make up for it and prevent dehydration. And when you eat, be sure to consume foods rich in the minerals sodium, potassium, magnesium, and calcium, or to at least take supplements to make sure you get what your body needs. Exact amounts depend on body size, of course, but the amounts of sodium, potassium, magnesium, and calcium you should get each day are 2,300-3,000 mg, 3,500-4,700 mg, 500 mg, and 1,250 mg respectively.

Not eating enough

It is hard to believe, but some people take up intermittent fasting and then don't eat enough when mealtime finally comes around. This is a bad idea because it will put your body in a state of calorie deprivation. This turns on starvation mode, which will slow your metabolism and reduce hormone activity. Intermittent fasting is not something to be used in conjunction with calorie deprivation. Make sure you eat until you are satiated at meal time.

Becoming obsessed

Fasting, in particular intermittent fasting, has many health benefits. However, these days, people can become obsessed with certain health programs and ideas about health and take things way too far. In fact, an example was in the news in the early spring of 2019. A woman in Israel took up a program of fruit juice fasting. The details aren't important— yes, fruit juice fasting is not technically fasting because she was still consuming calories—but the important thing was that she carried this out for longer and longer periods for a total of three weeks without stopping, and then became brain damaged from a lack of sodium. It is entirely ironic that a person would suffer from a lack of sodium in a world where excess sodium in processed foods is all around us. If you find yourself being more consumed with fasting, and tempted to push it past your limits, then reconsider and back off. You may even consider seeing a professional at that point because playing around too much with your body's nutritional system in excess is dangerous. Your body needs food, and fasting is only to be used as a tool, not a lifestyle.

Eating the wrong foods

The last mistake is one many will make. If you are only eating one meal per day, it is vital that you get a completely balanced meal. If you are doing keto, make sure you get plenty of leafy greens and avocado in your meals. Some people end up eating unbalanced meals and even snack on junk food. You don't want your body to be nutritionally deprived when you are using intermittent fasting.

Potential Risks and Downsides

The fact of the matter is that eating one meal per day is a minor risk to take unless you have some underlying major health problem. After all, you are getting plenty of food each day. That said, let's look at some of the risks:

Hypoglycemia

You may not be a diagnosed diabetic, or even have pre-diabetes; however, you may have problems with blood sugars (and hence be prone to developing pre-diabetes in the future). At present, you may not even be aware that you have this problem. As a result, being calorie deprived for a long time might put you at risk for hypoglycemia. There are a couple of ways you can deal with this. The first way is to ease into a fasting program gradually. The first day you decide to fast, don't go all in; instead, try out a 16:8 type fast first—to see how your body reacts to confining your food consumption to eight hours. After that, if all goes well, you can reduce the amount of time allotted toward eating, dropping down as time goes on, assuming no problems arise. A second thing to do is to invest in a blood sugar meter and track your blood sugars carefully. If you see your blood sugar dropping below 80 mg/dL, then you might want to back off. Note that this doesn't mean you need to give up fasting—fasting on a less rigorous level may be beneficial for you and set you up so that you can do one meal per day fasting later as your metabolism improves.

Problems exercising

Everyone is different. While many people will adjust to one-meal-a-day fasting quite easily, some people will find that it leaves them feeling weak and unenergetic. This may make it difficult to engage in exercise. If this happens to you, then you may consider limiting your fasting to a couple of days per week.

Mind fog

Some people experience heightened mental clarity while fasting. Others may actually experience the opposite. This may reflect how well your body adapts to ketosis and reduced blood sugars. As a result, you might experience brain fog.

Emotional problems

Some people will develop irritability, anxiousness, and other emotional problems. This might make it harder to get along with others.

While many of the problems listed above sound bad, and are potentially fatal when it comes to pursuing a program of intermittent fasting, don't let these problems kill an intermittent fasting program. Try fasting less frequently and using shorter fasting periods and then working your way up. If you need help, don't hesitate to discuss fasting with your doctor or mental health professional.

Frequently Asked Questions

Can I exercise?

Yes. If you are not a professional athlete, and you are pursuing a program of intermittent fasting that limits your fasting to a couple of days a week, you can choose to exercise on fasting days or non-fasting days—whichever works best for your body. Be sure to be careful if you have problems with hypoglycemia. Also, if you are a competitive athlete, you should probably eat a solid meal prior to competition.

I am a type 1 diabetic. Can I fast?

The short answer is maybe. Fasting is not a complete no-go for type 1 diabetics; however, you will need to discuss it in detail with your doctor and be sure to be under medical supervision when fasting.

What about those with pre-diabetes or type 2 diabetics?

Type 2 diabetics should also discuss fasting with their doctor. The main risk factor is hypoglycemia that may result from a failure to correctly adjust medications—something that will become necessary if you are fasting. This will not be an issue for pre-diabetics, although they may want to keep a close eye on their blood sugars. If you are following a keto-style low-carb diet before taking up fasting, this will be less of an issue because your body should already be adapted. In fact, fasting can go a long way toward curing or reversing both conditions.

What is refeeding syndrome, and do I need to worry about it?

Refeeding syndrome is rare, but it can happen in some people who have been without food intake when they start eating again. In short, serious complications can result from imbalances in minerals. A drop in phosphorous levels has been noted, and problems with edema or swelling can occur. However, refeeding syndrome is only a concern for people who go for an extended time without food. When it comes to fasting, the period is a minimum of five days and usually up to ten days in length. This is not a concern when it comes to people following a one-meal-a-day intermittent fasting plan because you will never be deprived of nutrients long enough for it to occur.

I feel dizzy when fasting. What is causing this?

When you are engaging in short-term fasting like a one-meal-a-day intermittent fasting program, more than likely dizziness is the result of dehydration. Try drinking more water to see if it helps. You can also make sure you are getting the proper amounts of minerals in your meals. If it continues, speak to your doctor to make sure that fasting has not revealed an underlying health condition.

When fasting, I develop constipation. What can I do about this?

If you develop constipation as a result of fasting, look toward your fiber and mineral intake. Magnesium can help alleviate constipation. Also, make sure you get plenty of fiber. Sources of fiber for keto dieters include avocados, leafy greens, nuts, and seeds.

Fasting gives me headaches. Any suggestions?

Try drinking more water and increasing your salt intake a bit.

Chapter 4 – Weight Loss with One Meal a Day

While fasting provides many benefits, most people are pursuing a program of fasting in the hopes of achieving weight loss. In this chapter, you will learn some of the ways that you can enhance weight loss using fasting techniques.

Starting Your One-Meal-A-Day Diet

First, the one-meal-a-day intermittent fasting program can work with any style of eating. You can incorporate it into virtually anything, including following the standard American diet as well as with veganism or vegetarian-style diets.

That said, the dieting approach that works the best by far is to incorporate it with a keto or ketogenic diet. The reason is simple: when you are following a ketogenic diet, you have laid down the groundwork that will help you get the most out of intermittent fasting. The fact of the matter is that ketosis is a vital part of fasting, and you are already in ketosis when following a keto or Atkins type diet. That saves hours, which can make your fasting more productive. A second benefit is simply put: the energy you get from a fatty meal is far more sustainable. A meal that incorporates more than 60 grams of carbohydrates is going to be one that gets burnt off quickly, causing increases in insulin levels and potentially leaving you feeling hungry hours after eating when a ketogenic meal simply will not.

It is important to be clear that vegans and vegetarians can follow a ketogenic diet. Ketogenic diets are great for meat eaters, but they do not require the consumption of meat. A vegan can make up the difference by consuming nuts, seeds, coconut, olives, and avocados.

That said, no matter what kind of diet you follow, there are some basic principles you can follow that will help you feel satisfied and get the most out of your fasting:

- *Make sure your meal is completely balanced nutritionally.*
- *Plan ahead.* One of the most important things is to make sure you don't undereat or engage in binge eating. You can work through this by knowing how many calories you want to consume each day, and then planning your meals to ensure this demand is met every time.
- *Pay special attention to minerals.* Remember to keep your digestion healthy and avoid heart palpitations, muscle cramps, and other mineral-related problems; you need to get sodium, potassium, calcium, and magnesium. You are going to need these minerals in adequate amounts, no matter how many calories you are consuming. Eating a salted avocado each day can go a long way toward meeting this goal.
- *Get adequate fiber.* It's important to get fiber to keep the digestion train rolling properly, but eating fiber also helps you feel full after eating. A good suggestion is to eat a handful of nuts to increase your fiber intake while also bulking up on important minerals.
- *Get lots of quality protein.* Not getting enough protein is a problem beginners often face when planning a one-meal-a-day diet. Going for a large protein source (a porterhouse steak, for example) is a good way to meet your daily

requirements. You can also add extras like cheese and nuts, which also include protein. Snack on some pork rinds. Add a second protein snack before your hour-long window is up, like some smoked salmon or cold cuts. A couple of slices of bacon can help too.

• *Eat lots of vegetables.* You can eat virtually unlimited amounts of leafy green vegetables. They contain fiber as well as plenty of nutrients. Consider stir-frying them in either olive oil or bacon grease. Meat eaters will find stir-frying in bacon grease helps up calories a bit while packing in the flavor.

When to Exercise

Exercise, including how much and when, is, of course, a personal preference; however, research has shown that people often end up preferring to exercise on fasting days. You may not find this to be the case initially, but as your body becomes better adjusted to intermittent fasting, you will find that it is easier to exercise during a fasting   period.

There is one diet pattern that is similar to a one-meal-a-day diet. This is called the "warrior diet", and it involves eating one large meal a day, and then exercising right before you eat. This is a good pattern to follow with this type of fasting because your body will be hungry for calories right after exercising, and it will help you accelerate your weight loss goals.

How Often to Follow a One-Meal-A-Day Fasting Plan

You can try to do a one-meal-a-day intermittent fasting plan daily, but the reality is that you are not going to get as many extra benefits from doing so as you might think. Most experts recommend doing your fasting two-three days per week.

Weight Loss Tips for Women

The main problem for women is often not getting enough protein. Stress centered around caregiver roles can also interfere with weight loss and making fasting difficult:

- *Eat adequate amounts of high-quality protein.* If you are following a keto diet and are not vegetarian or vegan, eat more steak and consume fatty fish like salmon and mackerel.
- *Don't avoid the fat.* Women have been conditioned by years of brainwashing to avoid eating fat. Fat does not make you fat; sugar does. Fat provides more sustainable long-term energy. Make sure you're getting enough—if you are fasting, this is especially important.
- *Drink more water.* A lack of water intake can cause problems when you are trying to incorporate fasting into your lifestyle.
- *Keep a food journal.* Knowing exactly what you're eating will help you pinpoint problems that arise when your goal is weight loss.
- *Get adequate amounts of sleep regularly.* A good night's sleep can go a long way toward keeping stress at bay.
- *Take up resistance training.* Weight lifting isn't just for bodybuilding men or professional athletes. Adding some weight training to your exercise routines will help you build lean muscle mass and lose weight more rapidly.
- *Get enough fiber.* Fiber helps you feel full and maintain healthy digestion. You can get fiber from green vegetables, avocados, nuts, and seeds.
- *Avoid yo-yo dieting.* One of the biggest problems with women is yo-yo dieting—a constant battle of dieting, losing weight and then gaining the weight back again when you stop dieting. A good way to avoid this is to avoid "dieting" in the first place. Pick a style of eating that works for you, and

incorporate it as a lifestyle change. Good examples are Keto, Paleo, or Vegan.

• *Stay away from fads.* The world is full of quick fixes that never really work. Fad diets might work for a short time, but before you know it, you'll tire of the diet and gain the weight back.

• *Avoid pills and potions.* There are many pills out there or "skinny teas" that promise rapid weight loss. The problem is that they are not healthy or sustainable.

• *Don't give in to everyone else's ideas of beauty.* We all want to look our best, but don't let that define who you are.

• *Set attainable goals.* Many people make goals in life that are too farfetched. For example, rather than making a goal of saving $100 a month, many people make a goal of "becoming a millionaire". When a goal is large and far off like that, you never take steps toward reaching it. Set goals that are easier to reach in small steps.

• *Avoid the calorie counting fallacy.* All of us, but women especially, have been brainwashed by decades of dietary disinformation. You are not a rabbit, so don't eat like one. Eat until you are full with satisfying foods that contain high-quality protein and fat, instead of counting every last calorie.

• *Limit refined carbohydrates.* If you are interested in intermittent fasting, the chances are that you're also practicing or looking into low-carb dieting. However, even if you aren't, you shouldn't eat refined carbohydrates. Instead, focus on whole grain foods. These are slower to digest and don't raise blood sugar as much.

Weight Loss Tips for Men

Men are often focused on losing belly fat. There are ways to decrease belly fat while also getting healthier like following a keto diet and adopting intermittent fasting:

• *Eat fewer carbs.* Recognize that belly fat often comes with metabolic syndrome. And metabolic syndrome is closely tied to problems metabolizing carbohydrates. If you have belly fat problems, then look into a low-carb diet.

• *Take up strength training.* If you aren't lifting weights now, add some strength training to your routine. You don't have to become a bodybuilder, but recognize that adding more muscle to your frame will rev up your metabolism and help you reduce body fat.

• *Have an awareness of heart disease.* It's important to note that heart disease impacts men and women, but it's going to impact men on average at younger ages. More recent studies are tying heart disease to the consumption of sugars. Adjust your diet accordingly.

• *Abdominal exercises may have their benefits, but they won't flatten your belly.* You'll build muscle by doing a lot of crunches and sit-ups, but if you aren't following a solid weight loss diet, you're not going to see six-pack abs magically appear. Weight loss seldom follows exercise alone.

• *Eat more veggies.* Many men avoid eating adequate amounts of veggies. Try developing a taste for them, as they have many needed micronutrients and additional benefits like providing a source of potassium and fiber. If you're not a fan of spinach, try frying it in bacon grease.

• *Don't always go for high-priced options.* Many men believe they can't follow a keto or Atkins diet because who can afford the daily steaks? The fact is: there are many low-priced options. Search for low-cost or cheap keto diets on the internet for suggestions.

• *Drink adequate amounts of water.* Just like for women, many men fail to drink enough water. If you're feeling fatigued, getting headaches or feeling dizzy while fasting, this may be part of the reason.

• *Get enough fiber.* The old joke is the man who has to read a magazine while using the bathroom. If that's your story, you're not getting enough fiber (and also probably not drinking enough water). Increase your intake of fiber through nuts, seeds, avocados, and green vegetables like spinach and broccoli. If you are doing a one-meal-a-day fasting plan, you'll want to make doubly sure that you get lots of green vegetables. Remember they pack on hardly any calories at all, so you can eat as many as you want. And try some celery too.

• *Keep a food journal.* This is important for everyone, but on average, it comes more naturally to women. Keeping a food journal is essential when you're trying to lose weight. It's important to know exactly what you're eating and when. Often when people begin keeping a food journal, they are surprised by the amounts of food they are really consuming.

• *Avoid sodas.* Studies have shown that even diet sodas can lead to weight gain. The reasons aren't clear at this point, but why not drink water instead?

• *Plan your grocery shopping.* If you live alone or your wife or husband isn't doing the shopping, plan your grocery shopping ahead of time. It can be too tempting walking around the store and seeing this and that food that looks tasty and can add to unnecessary calorie consumption.

• *Be careful when snacking.* One of the biggest mistakes you can make is thinking that because a snack is keto-compliant, that you can eat as much of it as you want. The reality is that pork rinds and other keto snacks still pack in calories and need to be enjoyed in moderation.

• *Listen to your body.* Don't always feel like you need to fill up a large plate and eat everything that's on it. When you feel full, stop.

• *Get aerobic exercise.* Weight training is great and essential for overall health, but don't neglect aerobic exercise.

• *Don't think you need to be "king of the hill".* Remember: you can get benefits from small amounts of things. When it comes to aerobic exercise, for example, you can get most of the benefit that exercise gives by simply walking 30 minutes a day. It's not necessary to run full blast for two hours.

• *Don't overdo it.* Many men overestimate their abilities or feel like they have to prove themselves. This need might express itself in a way that involves lifting more weight than they should or pushing their exercise too much (see the previous point). Stay within your abilities and grow slowly rather than feeling like you need to prove yourself.

Weight Loss Tips for Athletes

Athletes may have special needs when incorporating weight loss goals into their routines:

• *Test against performance to see how your new diet impacts your athletic performance.*

• *If a diet isn't working for you, don't be afraid to replace it with something else.*

• *Get adequate amounts of sleep.* Failure to get enough sleep can impair weight loss, in addition to keeping you from getting the most out of your body.

• *Make sure you properly fuel up before and after training.* Your body needs nutrients and calories for training. That is not the time to hold back on food consumption and don't fast during heavy training.

• *Avoid soda and junk food.* Even if soda is "diet", you should avoid it or at least consume in moderation.

• *Stay hydrated.* If you train heavily, being properly hydrated is that much more important.

• *Maintain protein intake while cutting back everything else.* Protein is important to keep up muscle strength. If you are trying to lose weight, keep protein constant in absolute terms while cutting back on other food items. When you've made your adjustments, then you should find that you're consuming a higher percentage of protein.

Weight Loss Tips for Vegans and Vegetarians

Vegans and vegetarians may think that certain dietary patterns are out of reach. In fact, the opposite is true. The only style of dieting that is out of reach is carnivore dieting, but any other diet can be adjusted for a vegan or vegetarian lifestyle:

- *Focus on high-fiber and high-protein foods.* More protein and fiber means less energy wasted on empty carbohydrates.

- *If you are interested in following a ketogenic diet, there are many high-fat plant foods you can use to play the role that meats do in a standard ketogenic diet.* Start with coconut and avocados. One single medium avocado contains 29 grams of fat with only small amounts of net carbohydrates. You can also eat nuts and seeds, which not only contain large amounts of fat but also protein.

- *Eat more fiber.*

- *Keep hydrated.* Not getting enough water can interfere with fasting and can slow weight loss, besides making you feel tired and irritable.

- *Eat more tofu and soy protein.* Fill yourself up with more tofu and fewer carbohydrates.

- *Eat a large amount of leafy greens.* Besides providing a large amount of nutrition, leafy greens also contain a large amount of fiber, which will help you feel full after eating.

- *Douse your food in olive oil.* Adding extra olive oil—and a lot of it—can add fat-based calories to your diet, which will help put you in a state of ketosis.

- *If you are vegetarian and not vegan, eat full-fat dairy.* Cheese can help provide protein and fat and can be very satisfying and filling. You can also get lots of fat-based calories from butter and cream.

• *Be careful with processed "meat substitutes".* Some are better than others. Consider "Beyond Meat" products which try to be more wholesome, rather than incorporate processed food.

• *Don't drink fruit juice.* It's really nothing more than sugar. If you want the benefits of fruit, eat it and don't drink it.

• *Stay away from sugar.* Whether or not you follow a keto diet, the verdict is in—sugar makes people fat. Eat whole grain carbohydrates, and avoid sugar and refined flours.

• *Eat beans.* The good thing about beans is they provide protein and fiber in one package. They fuel you with the protein you need while helping you feel satisfied with the extra boost from the fiber.

• *Stay away from food pyramids.* The sad truth is that they advocate styles of food consumption that make people gain, not lose, weight.

Chapter 5 – Your Brain on a Fast

How does fasting impact your brain, and what kind of energy and fuel does your brain need? People believe that the brain must have glucose to stay alive. While it is true that the brain should have some glucose—it needs about one-third of its energy from glucose—the myth that sugar powers the brain is just that: a myth. In fact, research is showing that running the brain on ketones actually helps it operate in a healthier state that impacts the very structure of the brain. Neural connections are increased and strengthened when the brain is fueled primarily by ketones. This has many practical effects, such as improving learning and memory, helping you stay focused and alert, and improving your moods.

While you can get these benefits by following a ketogenic diet, you don't need a ketogenic diet to do so—simply fasting will help you get these benefits. The reason is, of course, that while you are fasting—provided that you are not following a restricted-calorie type of "fast", you are fueling your body with ketones that are made from your body fat. In particular, the one-meal-a-day intermittent fasting method is well suited for this purpose. Along with 16:8 and 20:4 fasting methods, it is a type of fasting that you can incorporate into your lifestyle all the time. And since your fasting state is lengthened to 23 hours per day, you'll spend more time in ketosis than you will with the other methods (unless you are following a ketogenic diet; in that case, you're going to be in ketosis all the time).

In addition to getting the benefits that flow from fasting and being in ketosis through much of your day or all the time, several foods have direct benefits for the brain. In this chapter, we will have a look at several of these foods that you can incorporate into the meals you consume on your intermittent fasting plan. You will see that:

- Fasting actually helps the brain achieve a higher level of functioning by fueling it with ketones.
- You can magnify the effect by consuming foods that are known to help brain function.
- The ketogenic diet used to treat children who have epilepsy showed that ketones could enter the brain and improve neural function.

Finally, don't forget autophagy. In this chapter, we will be focusing on foods that will help the brain. However, autophagy also occurs during fasting and impacts the brain by clearing out harmful proteins and dead cells that can lead to horrible diseases like Alzheimer's and dementia.

Why Brain Food is Important

If you want to stay mentally fit and avoid problems like Alzheimer's, it is important to get the right brain food. First, it should be noted that the brain requires some glucose to function. That said, your brain does not have to rely strictly on blood sugar to function and at a high level. In fact, the brain can thrive and even do better when fueled with ketones.

Researchers discovered this back in the 1920s when they revealed that a ketogenic diet helped control epileptic seizures in children. For many years, if not decades, it wasn't recognized that a ketogenic diet might help the brain generally. Since that time, researchers have realized that a ketogenic diet helps maintain mood, helps people stay focused, improves mental clarity, and might help avoid problems like Alzheimer's and Parkinson's disease. Ketones help heal brain cells and help them function at the highest possible levels. It has also been demonstrated that ketones might help, slow, or stop the growth of deadly brain tumors, although more research is needed in this area. A fat-based diet has been shown to reduce the ups and downs of manic-depressive or bipolar disorder and has also been shown to help alleviate depression.

The brain can derive about 70% of its energy from ketones.

While ketogenic diets appear to help the brain, it is not strictly necessary to follow a ketogenic diet to get "brain food". In fact, better health for the brain can be attained by avoiding the highs and lows of fluctuating blood sugars. While your body will always work hard to keep the supply of glucose to the brain at adequate levels, fluctuating blood sugar levels can lead to irritability and anxiety, which obviously impact the emotional state of the brain. Fluctuating blood sugar levels also make it hard to focus and concentrate. For these reasons, a low-carb diet is recommended; however, if you tolerate it well, you can eat a carbohydrate-based diet, but make sure to include high-fiber foods, such as multigrain and whole fruits.

Omega-3 fats, in particular, seem to be important for proper and optimal brain function. These fats are found mainly in oily fish, and most Americans remain deficient in omega-3 fats. Other sources, which are important but less bioavailable, include walnuts and flax seeds. Omega-3 fats, and to a lesser extent omega-6 oils, which are found in foods like sunflower seeds, may help to strengthen synaptic connections in the brain.

Any food that is rich in antioxidants will help with brain health. Oxidation processes, which happen during normal metabolism, damage cells throughout the body, including brain cells. Foods rich in antioxidants like spinach, carrots, and blueberries can help protect brain cells from this type of damage.

Here is a list of important brain foods:

• *Oily fish:* Eat oily fish at least twice a week, and more if possible. Oily fish includes the omega-3 fats discussed above in large amounts. Good examples of oily fish include salmon, sardines, mackerel, trout, herring, anchovies, arctic char, and barramundi. If you don't like eating fish, consider a supplement. The problem with supplements is making sure that you're getting adequate doses and that they contain the right mix of fats. Aim for a brand that lets you get a gram a day or more of actual omega-3 fats, which may be listed on the label as DHA and EPA. Omega-3 fats help maintain the structural integrity of nerve cells and also help maintain a healthy level of blood flow to the brain. Omega-3 fats also reduce inflammation, and studies show that reduced inflammation in the body helps brain health.

• *Dark Chocolate:* It turns out that certain compounds called flavonoids help protect brain tissue. One tasty way to increase your brain food consumption is to eat some dark chocolate.

• *Blueberries and blackberries:* These tasty fruits are not only low in blood sugar but contain many phytonutrients that help reduce inflammation and help brain cells communicate with one another.

• *Nuts and seeds:* These food items contain healthy fats in the form of omega-3 fatty acids and monounsaturated fats. Unfortunately, the effectiveness of omega-3 oils in nuts is far less than that found in fish because the compounds are less bioavailable to humans. Extra processing is necessary to get the omega-3 benefits. However, the monounsaturated fats in nuts and seeds are very strong when it comes to reducing inflammation, and so eating a daily dose of nuts and seeds can help you achieve better brain health.

• *Whole grains:* While you may be avoiding them if you are on a keto diet, if you are not following a low-carb eating plan, you should be eating whole grains. In addition to leading to fewer blood sugar spikes, which hurt the brain, whole grains contain vitamin E, which has been shown to be important for brain health.

• *Avocados*: If you are on a keto diet, avocadoes are your friend. They are literally packed with inflammation-fighting monounsaturated fats.

• *Coffee:* A cup of joe can help you maintain mental sharpness. And the effect is real; it's no illusion. Coffee helps strengthen nerve signals, which is why it makes you feel awake.

Brain Fog – Foods to Avoid

The biggest culprit that contributes to brain fog is fluctuating blood sugars. So you want to avoid foods that will lead to blood sugar spikes, which may give the sensation of temporary mental clarity. However, the benefits are short-lived. When the blood sugar levels crash, then you will lose the ability to concentrate and operate at peak efficiency.

Any food that leads to clogged blood vessels is to be avoided. In the case of the brain, you are concerned with reduced blood flow in your jugular veins, which are two large blood vessels in your neck. You also want to avoid blockages in any arteries supplying the brain. For the most part, sugars and refined carbohydrates are the foods to avoid here. Over time, sugar consumption can lead to metabolic syndrome, higher triglycerides, and small LDL particles that are prone to sticking to arterial walls. This can lead to blockages that not only cause heart attacks but can reduce blood flow to the brain. In a best-case scenario, there is simply reduced blood flow to the brain, which, over time, may cause mental fog to turn into a form of dementia. In a worst-case scenario, you may have a stroke leading to catastrophic results.

Alcohol is something that comes to mind here, as well. It really is a double-edged sword. When consumed in moderation, alcohol can be healthy and, in particular, leads to better brain health. In moderate amounts, alcohol also helps thin the blood, leading to secondary benefits that accrue because you have better blood flow to the brain. This works fine up to a couple of drinks per day; however, beyond that, you may run into many health problems. One problem you might have is too much blood thinning, which can even lead to bleeding in the brain and death. So alcohol can be consumed but in moderation.

Fish that is high in mercury could also cause problems if consumed in high amounts. Two common fish varieties that are high in mercury are tuna and swordfish. Mercury has long been associated with mental decline as well as with mental illness. Of course, if you are going to develop problems from mercury as an adult, you are going to have to consume large amounts of fish. In most cases, if you are eating tuna once a week (say) and the occasional piece of swordfish, then mercury is not going to be an issue. Pregnant and nursing mothers should avoid mercury containing fish, however, since it has a strong impact on early brain development. Fish like sardines and trout are low in mercury.

Soda and artificial sweeteners. Soda should be avoided, mainly because of the fluctuations in blood sugar that may result. Diet sodas containing artificial sweeteners should be consumed in moderation.

Refined carbohydrates. Earlier, we noted that whole grains are better for the brain. The converse holds true as well—refined carbohydrates are bad for the brain and should be avoided. Don't eat white flour or white rice, or any food that has a high glycemic index.

Also, avoid foods that are made out of refined carbs like white bread and any pasta that is not a whole grain variety.

A special note: Many websites go around promoting the idea that red meat is bad for brain health. This is false and is largely due to old-school notions about saturated fat and cholesterol. It has been found in recent years that there is no scientific relationship between red meat and heart attacks, stroke, or clogged arteries. So it is safe to consume red meat when it comes to brain health and, in fact, may even be desirable.

Practical Tips for Increasing Mental Clarity and Boosting Brain Power

Here are some practical tips for increasing mental clarity and brain power that you can use in addition to making the right dietary choices:

- *Get lots of exercise.* It has been repeatedly demonstrated that staying physically fit is good for the brain and the body. You can increase your mental clarity by getting good, routine, aerobic exercise.
- *Get lots of sleep.* Failure to get adequate sleep takes a strong toll on the brain. In fact, when you sleep, your body is hard at work, cleaning out the junky, clogging proteins associated with Alzheimer's disease from your brain. Lack of sleep leads to mental fogginess now and may lead to dementia down the road.
- *Do crossword puzzles.* Crossword puzzles are a great way to challenge your brain without enrolling at a university. They help strengthen memory and sharpen concentration.
- *Learn a language.* Learning a language, and in fact learning anything, helps with brain plasticity. If you are an adult, you can learn at your own pace, but learning a second language has been shown to have multiple benefits.
- *Practice sharpening your focus.* You can boost brain power by learning how to shut off outside distractions.
- *Deal with stress effectively.* Stress makes it hard to concentrate, and the heightened stress hormones that accompany it may cause long-term brain damage.
- *Don't drink alcohol excessively.* We already noted that excessive alcohol consumption could lead to bleeding inside the brain. Even if you don't drink to those levels, heavy

drinking kills brain cells. You only have one brain in this life; killing brain cells is probably not something you want to encourage. This advice pertains to any drug that you can take as well, not just alcohol.

• *Do breathing exercises.* This helps you relax and focus. It also helps get your mind and body in tune.

• *Learn to write with your opposite hand.* If you try it for the first time, it will be more challenging than you expect. You can help wire new brain circuits by learning to write with the opposite hand you usually use.

• *Practice mindfulness.* Like getting a good night's sleep, mindful meditation can help relax the mind and heal the brain.

• *Yoga.* Yoga has been shown to help relax the brain, improve mental focus, and improve the mind-body connection.

Fasting and the Brain

Research in animal models has shown that fasting directly benefits the brain. In particular, fasting promotes the formation of more neural connections, which boosts brain power. More than likely, these effects come about from the dependence by the brain on ketones for most of its fuel while in the fasted state. The brain cell growth happens in between fasted states, although it is actually caused by fasting (via the use of ketones as fuel). Animal models testing fasting have found that animals who fast have more alertness and better learning and memory capabilities. While these types of tests have not been done extensively in humans, they are consistent with what people report who use fasting as part of their lifestyle.

Chapter 6 – Guilt-Free Wellness on a Fast

In this era of downright obsession with health and eating, it is important to adopt a guilt-free attitude toward food. Practical steps can be taken to ensure that you are following a healthy lifestyle that is suitable for your body type and family history, but you should not let food, nutrition, and eating become an obsession. One advantage that you will find you gain by adopting a one-meal-a-day intermittent fasting routine is that you will spend less time thinking about food and nutrition. In the beginning, it will be a little difficult as you battle the urge to eat during all waking hours, but when your body has completely adjusted to this new way of taking in food, you will find that overall food plays less of a role in your life than it used to.

Stop Shaming Yourself

We live during a time of nearly unimaginable plenty, and this has brought many people into the twin plagues of obesity and chronic disease. We are surrounded by ample amounts of food while advised by experts to eat fewer calories. This has caused many people many problems. While we strongly recommend a limited fasting program for your overall lifestyle in order to promote optimal health, whether it is the one-meal-a-day fasting program or 16:8 or 20:4 fasting, it's important not to let it take over your life.

Remember the woman who got so obsessed with following a fruit juice fast that she suffered irreversible brain damage from a lack of sodium. You don't want to become too obsessed with healthy eating and fasting that you follow her down a path like that.

One reason that so many people do become obsessed with health and healthy eating is that we are victims of shame. You should feel no shame in adopting a healthy lifestyle, which may include a specialized diet, or not, and intermittent fasting. Instead, feel proud of yourself for taking control of your health.

Another thing to avoid is shaming yourself because of your food choices. If you decide to follow a specialized diet, you can do so but do it because you want to, not because other people are saying meat is unhealthy or carbs are evil. However, it is important to realize that although keto and low-carb diets can help you maintain a state of ketosis, it's not necessary to adopt any specialized type of diet to benefit from intermittent fasting. Some people get great results eating whatever they want while also following an intermittent fasting diet. So, if you don't want to become a vegan, carnivore, or follow keto, you don't have to in order to achieve great results.

One of the issues that have arisen with the proliferation of specialized diets is guilt. The guilt can come from the inability to follow the strict requirements of specialized diets that require you to cut out entire food groups or tasty snacks. It is important to realize that you can get massive benefits from intermittent fasting without following the latest diet fad, and you should be able to eat what you like without worrying about what others think or whether or not the food you like fits in with the latest banned food list or not.

The bottom line is that you can change your diet if you want to before taking up intermittent fasting, or you can keep your diet if you don't want to change it. Intermittent fasting will benefit you either way.

Forbidden food can be the sweetest. So, if you have problems with avoiding certain types of foods, you can avoid focusing on a specialized diet and use intermittent fasting alone to help you with your weight loss needs.

Practical, Guilt-Free Wellness Tips

The following tips will help you maintain guilt-free fasting:

- *Avoid calorie restriction.* This can lead to low energy levels. Get enough calories for an entire day.
- *Build up slowly.* Start with two meals splitting your calories, then work toward eating all of your calories in one meal.
- *Be patient.* See how eating various foods impacts your weight in the context of doing intermittent fasting. Some people may be able to tolerate a wider variety of foods than others. Pick a diet that works for you and realize that many people achieve large amounts of weight loss without doing any dieting at all by using intermittent fasting.
- *The longer you fast, the longer your body is burning fat with lower levels of insulin.*
- *Eat natural whole foods for your best state of health.*
- *As long as you're losing weight and feeling good, eat what works for you.* People have found many different ways to lose weight, from keto dieting to even eating junk food in prescribed caloric amounts.
- *If you crave something, eat it, and eat as much as you want as long as its during your one-hour feeding period.*
- *Don't pay attention to day-to-day fluctuations on the scale.* Your weight can be declining over a long-term period, but seesawing over short-term day-to-day fluctuations may give a false picture. For example, when you eat a high-sodium

meal, you can retain water weight, making it look like you've gained weight.

- *Keep protein intake relatively high, so that you don't lose any muscle mass.*

- *Eat enough fats so that you'll avoid slowing down your metabolism.*

Fun, Guilt-Free Meal Plans

When following a one-meal-a-day diet start from three principles:

- *Make sure you consume an adequate level of calories to get you through one full day.* A one-meal-a-day fasting program is not a calorie deprivation diet.

- *Have everything you are going to eat ready in front of you before you eat.*

- *Eat whatever you want.* This means you can eat anything if specialized dieting is not your thing. If you are following any diet, you can eat whatever foods are permitted on that diet in adequate quantities to satisfy your daily caloric needs.

- *Work up to a one meal per day lifestyle.* You're not going to be used to it at first, and your stomach might not handle it. Begin by compressing to two meals a day and shortening your feeding window.

Here are some fun guilt-free ideas to include in your meals:

- *Break up your eating into multiple meals all consumed within one hour.* That makes eating a lot of food over a short period easier.

- *Eat a giant bowl of salad.* Remember: you're only eating once per day, so if you would eat two salads a day, make enough for two salads and eat all of it. Fill your salad with anything you enjoy, from spinach to tomatoes and sunflower seeds, with lots of dressing.

- *Eat two chicken thighs with skin on, or a basket of chicken wings flavored to taste.*

- *Mash up an avocado with some salsa and pink Himalayan salt to make a good homemade guacamole, then dive in with some blue corn chips.*
- *Eat some fried chicken.* You can eat all you want on this kind of diet up to your total daily caloric limit. If you feel like eating more, feel free to do so as long as it fits within the time window.
- *Alternate between steak, pork, chicken, and fish to keep your meals fresh and interesting.*
- *Balance is the key to your overall meal plan.* What determines what balance is right will be your overall lifestyle, but you will want to include every food group in adequate proportions to balance your meal.
- *Eating sandwiches is a good way to get in many calories and include multiple food groups.*
- *Eat spaghetti and meatballs with lots of cheese.*
- *Top your meal off with a chocolate bar or some ice cream.*

Appendix – Sample Meal Plans

Now let's examine the basics of the one-meal-a-day food plan. The important point here is you have to really make your one meal per day count, as it is going to be the only time that you are taking in food and nutrients. So you want to make sure you get a balanced meal that provides enough calories while providing nutritional benefits.

Begin by figuring out how many calories you will need based on your gender and body size. Some smaller framed women, for example, will only eat 1,800-2,000 calories per day, while some active men may range from 3,000 all the way up to 4,000 calories consumed in a single meal.

- *Eat large amounts of high-fiber vegetables.* Spinach, arugula, kale, broccoli, cucumber, and zucchini are good to include. In terms of quantity, these foods should form the biggest portion of your meal. Other good vegetables include celery, asparagus, cauliflower, and cabbage.

- *Next, consider including large amounts of fats and oils.* Avocados are excellent and can be included in any diet, such as vegan, keto, or paleo. Avocados not only provide many calories from fat, but they also provide anti-inflammatory oils, along with large amounts of potassium and magnesium. Also, include a daily serving of nuts and seeds. Butter and cheese can also be included.

• *Protein should be consumed with oil.* Find out the daily recommended amount of protein for your body size and type and make sure you get enough in your meal (you only have one meal per day, so make sure you get everything). You can eat multiple sources of protein in your single meal. Good sources of protein include grass-fed beef, free-range skin-on chicken, eggs, fish, and seafood—salmon, sardines, tuna, and mackerel are excellent choices. You can also consume limited amounts of bacon and some processed meats. Vegans can get protein from nuts and seeds as well as from beans and legumes. Garbanzo beans and kidney beans are excellent protein sources for vegans (and anyone else for that matter). You can also add to your diet by consuming vegetarian or vegan shake mixes made out of soy or other vegetable-based proteins.

• Next is carbs. If you are following keto or Atkins style eating, you will limit your carbs to that found in vegetables. Tomatoes are also a good choice. If you are following a paleo type diet, your options are more open and include root vegetables like sweet potato, carrot, turnip, and even the occasional regular potato and peas.

• Next, we have items that can be consumed in smaller amounts, depending on taste. This includes fruits and berries, yogurt, and milk products.

It is important to note that the one-meal-a-day intermittent fasting diet is not really a "diet" at all, and you can follow any style of eating that suits your needs and preferences. Therefore, there really aren't specific rules on what to eat or consume. The only rules to follow are:

• Each day, go 23 hours without eating.
• Consume all foods within a one-hour window.
• Make sure you get enough daily calories that you would normally eat.

- Don't skimp on calories—this will actually cause you to lose less weight.

- Make sure you get all the nutrition your body needs, including adequate fat and nutrients.

- Pay special attention to protein and make sure you consume adequate levels. Since you are only eating one meal per day, you will probably want to eat multiple sources of protein in your one sitting.

- If you are not avoiding carbs, stick to whole grains, but you can eat rice, pasta, bread, quinoa, couscous, and fruits like bananas and oranges in any amount you desire.

Conclusion

Thank you for taking the time to read *One-Meal-a-Day Intermittent Fasting: How You Can Activate Autophagy, Lose Weight, and Increase Your Mental Clarity Without Feeling Guilty About Eating Delicious Food.* It should have been informative, educational, and provided you with all of the tools you need to achieve your fasting goals.

People have been fasting since the dawn of time. However, the powers of fasting, which were recognized by the great minds of history and by the great religious traditions, were lost in modernity as the 20th century developed. It has only been in the last five-ten years when the healing benefits of fasting have been rediscovered.

In addition to realizing that fasting is a healing activity, people have discovered that there are many different ways that you can fast. It is now possible for a person to enjoy fasting while choosing a personally suitable method. You can fast for as long as you like or only do it for sixteen hours—the choice is up to you.

Fasting fits in best with a low-carb diet, with keto taking the award for the most suitable diet. However, you can utilize fasting with virtually any kind of eating, even with the standard American diet. People have been shown to get many health benefits when fasting while eating whatever they want during fed periods. However, that is not recommended. To achieve optimal health, you should also incorporate a healthy diet into your lifestyle and not use fasting as an attempt to undo the damage done by eating the refined carbohydrates and junk food found in the standard American diet.

There are many benefits of fasting, including:

- Weight loss
- Increased mental clarity
- Decreased insulin levels and increased insulin sensitivity
- Lower blood sugar levels
- Reduced blood pressure
- Autophagy
- Increased lifespan and anti-aging effects

The one-meal-a-day intermittent fasting diet lets you get these health benefits and more without the pain and risk of longer-term fasting programs. Best of luck on your health journey, and be sure to consult with a doctor before making any major changes to your diet or lifestyle.

Check out another book by Elizabeth Moore

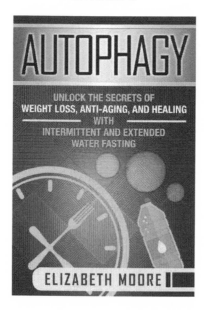